THE ULTIMATE VISUAL GUIDE TO
HAIRSTYLES

A GALLERY OF 160 GREAT LOOKS FOR EVERY KIND OF HAIR TYPE AND LENGTH

THE ULTIMATE VISUAL GUIDE TO
HAIRSTYLES

A GALLERY OF 160 GREAT LOOKS FOR EVERY KIND OF HAIR TYPE AND LENGTH

Learn stylist's secrets for beautiful hair with essential information on haircare and hairstyling, illustrated in over 290 inspiring photographs

NICKY POPE

This edition is published by Southwater, an imprint of Anness Publishing Ltd, Blaby Road, Wigston, Leicestershire LE18 4SE; www.southwaterbooks.com; www.annesspublishing.com

If you like the images in this book and would like to investigate using them for publishing, promotions or advertising, please visit our website www.practicalpictures.com for more information.

Publisher: Joanna Lorenz
Senior Editor: Lucy Doncaster
Project Editor: Dan Hurst
Designer: Simon Daley
Jacket Designer: Lisa Tai
Illustrator: Vanessa Card
Production Controller: Bessie Bai

ETHICAL TRADING POLICY
At Anness Publishing we believe that business should be conducted in an ethical and ecologically sustainable way, with respect for the environment and a proper regard to the replacement of the natural resources we employ.

As a publisher, we use a lot of wood pulp in high-quality paper for printing, and that wood commonly comes from spruce trees. We are therefore currently growing more than 750,000 trees in three Scottish forest plantations: Berrymoss (130 hectares/320 acres), West Touxhill (125 hectares/305 acres) and Deveron Forest (75 hectares/185 acres). The forests we manage contain more than 3.5 times the number of trees employed each year in making paper for the books we manufacture.

Because of this ongoing ecological investment programme, you, as our customer, can have the pleasure and reassurance of knowing that a tree is being cultivated on your behalf to naturally replace the materials used to make the book you are holding.

Our forestry programme is run in accordance with the UK Woodland Assurance Scheme (UKWAS) and will be certified by the internationally recognized Forest Stewardship Council (FSC). The FSC is a non-government organization dedicated to promoting responsible management of the world's forests. Certification ensures forests are managed in an environmentally sustainable and socially responsible way. For further information about this scheme, go to www.annesspublishing.com/trees

A CIP catalogue record for this book is available from the British Library.

Previously published as part of a larger volume, *The Professional's Illustrated Guide to Haircare & Hairstyles.*

PUBLISHER'S NOTE
Although the advice and information in this book are believed to be accurate and true at the time of going to press, neither the authors nor the publisher can accept any legal responsiblity or liability for any errors or omissions that may be made nor for any inaccuracies nor for any harm or injury that comes about from following instructions or advice in this book. All electrical equipment should be used with caution and should never be left unattended.

Bracketed terms are intended for American readers.

AUTHOR'S NOTE
Special thanks for their encouragement and help to Louise Wood and Susan Pope for being my second eyes, and to Tim Frisby for getting me started. I'm grateful to Lucy Doncaster for being unflappable, patient and very good at what she does.

CONTENTS

Introduction

How you wear your hair and the way it makes you look and feel is incredibly important. Whether hair is groomed, worn loose and casual, or even remains unkempt, do remember that its look, colour, texture and style is all part of your individuality.

Although genetic factors determine the type, natural colour and texture of your hair, the rest is down to you. The way you live your life, your state of health and your haircare regime will impact on the overall appearance of your hair and its capacity to shine, move and look vital.

For many centuries women all over the world have been changing the colour of their hair, originally using dyes made from natural sources such as henna and, in modern times, from chemical colourants, although natural dyes are still popular.

The desire to curl or wave straight hair or smooth out natural curls is also pervasive in most cultures, and as new techniques and tools develop, the power of a hairstyle to entirely change a person's look becomes ever more apparent – it's almost a magical way to reinvent an identity.

It's no surprise, then, that so many women spend time and energy in getting their hair to look a certain way, and stay like that. From hours in the bathroom, washing, fixing and styling hair, to countless trips to the salon for cut, colour

Above Learn how to wear accessories, hats and ornaments in a way that balances your face shape and works with your dress style.

and waving services, it seems that hair and hairdressing is bigger business than ever. But with so much advice available, so many products and such a choice of hairstyling tools and equipment spilling off shelves in the shops, it's not quite so easy to figure out what to do for the best! How will you know what style is right for you? How should you care for your hair and makes sure every day is a good hair day?

The answers lie in understanding your hair and learning to manage it well, and this beautiful book tells everything you will ever need to know about your hair, from basic care to styling and dressing it yourself so that you can be confident that your hair looks fantastic each time you step out of the door.

The book opens with basic information about healthy hair, including guidance to help you assess your own hair, its texture and type, and understand how to tackle problems in the short- and long-term so that you will be better able to keep it in great condition. By looking at the structure of different hair types, and considering the impact of diet, lifestyle and different care regimes, you will learn

Left Regard your hair as an asset. Shiny, healthy hair dressed to suit your individual look is an important part of your identity and personal style.

Above Choosing which hair products to use can be daunting. Develop a routine and stick with products that work for your hair.

what to do for your particular type. Problems that occur naturally or arise through medical illness can be tackled and we explain how to recognize various conditions and what action to take.

Good haircare regimes are essential to looking fabulous and we teach you how to establish good routines, cope with wayward or damaged hair, and how to use both manufactured and natural products to look after your hair properly. This is especially important as your hair

Below Experimenting with different hair styles and colours allows you to reinvent your look on a regular basis, or create an impact for a special occasion.

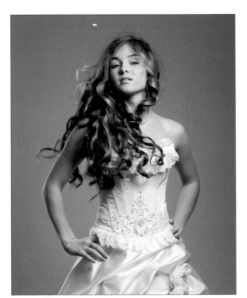

ages and its condition and appearance changes, or when external factors such as the sun, wind, heat and pollution have an impact on your hair. We have a happy holiday guide to enable you to provide the correct care for your hair in all weathers.

There then follows a chapter on successful styling, including advice and ideas on how to select a salon that's right for you, and what to expect when you get there – from levels of service to understanding what your hairdresser is talking about.

There is useful information on the which styles will suit your face shape, and on choosing a style that will suit your lifestyle. One of the most important factors to consider when choosing a new style is versatility, and it is a good idea to consider the options your new cut will give you to change your look for work and play. This section gives you advice on this and examines the other factors to consider before commiting to a new style.

Processes such as colouring, perming and straightening are also demystified, with advice on how to get the best results both at home and from professional salon services.

Finally, a series of illustrated style galleries will help to give you the inspiration to try something different.

Successful styling comes from picking a cut to suit your look, and it is important that you can maintain it with ease. From short to mid-length or long, and straight to curly, our pages of more than 160 styles will give you plenty of ideas.

Hair is a good indicator of your health and state of mind, so enjoy its potential and bring out the best in yourself. Learn to love your hair and wear it with style.

Right Looking after your hair should be an integral part of your beauty routine. Put aside dedicated time to pamper yourself, a little self-indulgence will leave you feeling great and looking fabulous.

Above Develop a good realtionship with a professional stylist; it is important that you feel confident enough to give honest feedback and trust your hairdresser with dramatic changes.

Healthy hair

Beautiful, shining hair can and should make you look and feel great. It is a versatile fashion accessory, and you can change its colour, texture, shape and length to suit your mood and personal style. In order to maintain optimum health of your hair, however, you need to know what impact environmental stresses will have on its condition and shine, including the damage caused by over-exposure to sun, wind, air-conditioning or central heating. It's equally important to maintain a balanced diet and good haircare and styling routines to ensure your hair is your natural crowning glory.

What is hair?

Understanding the structure of hair and how it forms will give you a better grasp of how to achieve healthy hair. Armed with this knowledge, you can go on to improve the condition of your own hair and pinpoint any particular problems you may have.

A human hair consists mainly of a protein called keratin, which is also found in your nails. It also contains some moisture as well as trace metals and minerals that are found in the rest of the body. The visible part of the hair, called the shaft, is dead tissue: the only living part of the hair is its root, called the dermal papilla, which lies snugly below the surface of the scalp in a tube-like depression known as the hair follicle. The dermal papilla is made up of cells that are fed by the bloodstream in the skin.

Each hair consists of three layers. The outer layer, or cuticle, is the hair's protective shield and has tiny overlapping scales, rather like tiles on a roof. When the cuticle scales lie flat and neatly overlap the hair feels silky-soft and looks glossy. If the cuticle scales have been physically or chemically damaged or broken, however, the hair will be dull and brittle and will tangle easily.

Under the cuticle lies the cortex, which is made up of fibre-like cells that give hair its strength and elasticity. The cortex also contains the pigment called melanin, which gives hair its natural colour.

At the centre of the hair is the medulla, consisting of soft keratin cells interspersed with spaces. The function of the medulla is not known, but it may carry nutrients and other substances to the cortex and cuticle. This could explain why hair is affected so rapidly by changes in general health.

Why does hair shine?

Hair's natural shine is a result of sebum, which is an oil composed of waxes and fats that contains a natural antiseptic that helps fight infection. Sebum is produced by the sebaceous glands present in the dermis (the skin). These glands are linked to the hair follicles and release sebum into them. As a lubricant, sebum gives an excellent protective coating to the entire hair shaft, smoothing the cuticle scales and helping hair retain its natural moisture and elasticity.

The smoother the surface of the cuticle, the more light will be reflected from the hair and, therefore, the higher the level of hair shine will be. This is why it is more difficult to obtain a shine on curly hair than on straight hair, as on curly hair the cuticle isn't so smooth. Under certain circumstances, such as excessive hormonal activity, the sebaceous glands produce too much sebum, and the result is oily hair. Conversely, if too little sebum is produced, the hair will be dry.

The growth cycle of hair

Hair goes through three stages of growth: the anagen phase when it actively grows, which lasts between two to four years; the catagen, or transitional phase, when the hair stops growing but cellular activity continues in the papilla, and which lasts 90–120 days; and the telogen, or resting phase, when growth stops completely. During the telogen phase there is no further growth or activity at the papilla; eventually the old hair is pushed out by the new growth and the cycle begins all over again.

At any given time, about 93 per cent of an individual's hair is in the anagen phase, 1 per cent is in the catagen phase, and 6 per cent is in the telogen phase. Scalp hair, which reacts to hormonal stimuli just like hair on the rest of the

Sweat duct   Hair shaft

Touch receptor

Erector pilli muscle

Blood supply

Sweat gland

Epidermis

Dermis

Sebaceous gland

Hair follicle

Dermal papilla

Subcutaneous fat

Left *The structure of the skin is complex, comprising many elements, including hair follicles, dermal papillae and sebaceous glands.*

Did you know?

- *Hair grows about 1cm/½in per month.*
- *A single strand lives for up to seven years.*
- *If a person never had their hair cut it could grow to a length of about 107cm/42in before falling out.*
- *Women have more hair than men.*
- *Hair grows faster in the summer and during sleep.*
- *Hairs grow fastest between the ages of 16 and 24 years.*
- *Between the ages of 40 and 50 women tend to lose about 20 per cent of their hair.*
- *Hair becomes drier with age.*

body, is genetically programmed to repeat its growth cycle 24–25 times during the average person's lifetime.

Above *The hair's cuticle is formed by overlapping scales that need to lie close and flat to allow hair to shine. Here, they are roughened, indicating brittle and dull hair.*

Above *The central section of the hair is called the medulla, consisting of softer keratin. Surrounding this is the cortex, which gives hair its strength and elasticity, and the cuticle.*

The importance of diet

Like the rest of the body, the health and condition of hair is dependent upon a consistently good diet, which ensures it is supplied with all the necessary nutrients for sustained growth and health.

Regular exercise is also important as it promotes good blood circulation, which

Below *Regular exercise and good grooming routines will help keep your hair healthy.*

in turn ensures that vital oxygen and nutrients are transported to the hair root via the blood.

Poor eating habits and lack of regular exercise are soon reflected in the state of our hair, and even a minor case of short-term ill-health can often make the hair look limp and lacklustre. Although there are many products and supplements on the market that claim to improve the

condition of hair, if you eat a balanced diet containing plenty of fresh, raw ingredients, including fruit and vegetables, you shouldn't need to take any supplementary vitamins to promote healthy hair growth and condition.

Drinking plenty of water (between six and eight glasses a day), herbal teas and unsweetened fruit juice will keep you hydrated and your hair looking good.

Tips for healthy hair

- *Cut down on tea and coffee if you can – these are powerful stimulants that act on the nervous, respiratory and cardiovascular systems, increasing the excretion of water and important nutrients. They also hamper the absorption of minerals that are crucial for hair health.*
- *Alcohol dilates blood vessels and so helps increase blood flow to the tissues, including the scalp. However, alcohol is antagonistic to several minerals and vitamins that are vital for healthy hair, so it should only be consumed in moderation.*
- *Regular exercise stimulates the circulatory system, encouraging a healthy blood supply to all cells and nourishing and helping to regenerate and repair.*
- *Any type of medication can potentially affect the condition of your hair. If you notice any dramatic change in its condition, such as significant hair loss or thinning, then you should tell your doctor as soon as possible.*

The ages of hair

As our bodies grow older, so too does our hair, and this affects the way it is produced and in what quantities, as well as its texture and type. It is important, therefore, that care regimes are adjusted accordingly depending on your age and stage.

The baby and child

A baby's hair characteristics are determined from the very moment of conception. By the 16th week of pregnancy the foetus will be covered with lanugo, a downy body hair that is usually shed before or around birth. The first hair appears on the baby's head by around the 20th week of pregnancy and it is at this time that the pigment, melanin, which will determine the colour of the hair, is first produced.

A few weeks after birth, the baby's original hair begins to fall out or is rubbed off. The new hair is quite different from the initial downy mass, so a baby born with blonde, wispy curls might have dark straight hair by the age of six months.

Cradle cap, which appears as thick, yellow scales in patches over the scalp, can be a common problem at this age.

This is the result of a natural build-up of skin cells and can be gently loosened by rubbing a little baby oil on to the scalp at night and washing it off in the morning. This may need to be repeated for several days until all the scales have been removed.

Children's hair is normally in beautiful condition and is best cut and styled simply. At the onset of puberty, however, this may all change, and many young people experience oily hair and skin for the first time as a result of hormone changes.

Ageing

As we grow older our hair changes, and by the age of 30 to 40 years old some hair will grow without melanin, so be colourless. The production of melanin is governed by genetic factors, and the best indication of when your hair will become grey is the age at which your parents' hair lost its colour.

Apart from giving hair its colour, melanin also helps to soften and make each strand more flexible. This is why white hair tends to become wirier and coarser in texture. The ageing hair also loses elasticity and becomes rougher as the scalp produces less sebum.

Because the texture changes, the hair is inclined to pick up dust and smoke from the atmosphere, so it soon appears discoloured and dirty-looking. Mineral deposits from chlorinated water can give white hair a greenish tinge. Chelating, clarifying, or purifying shampoos will help to strip this build-up from the hair.

To counteract the dryness associated with ageing hair, use specially formulated richer shampoos and conditioning products on a regular basis. In addition, weekly intensive treatments are essential to counteract moisture loss.

Above The amount of hair and hair type of a newborn child does not necessarily indicate how their hair will be as they age.

Right White and grey hair needs special care and products to combat dryness and restore vitality and elasticity.

Pregnancy and post-natal hair

During pregnancy, many women feel their hair often looks its best. This is perhaps because the hormonal changes stop hair falling out at the same rate so it feels thicker. Pregnant women also have more blood coursing through their veins than usual and as it circulates it feeds the scalp to help hair become healthier. However, after the birth or after breast-feeding ceases, this thick, glossy extra hair can be lost at what may seem to many an alarming rate. What appears to be excessive hair loss is therefore simply a postponement of a natural occurrence, a condition that is known as post-partum alopecia.

Another more significant problem that may occur during pregnancy and while breast-feeding is caused by a depletion in the protein content of the hair, causing it to become drier and more brittle. Combat this by frequently using an intensive conditioning treatment.

In some women, pregnancy can affect the hair type, changing curly hair to straight or vice versa. It may then revert back to its prior condition once the baby is born, although occasionally it does not.

There's a view that it's best to avoid perming during pregnancy because the hair is in an altered state and the result can be unpredictable. However, a new colour can give your hair a lift.

The menopause and beyond

Many women report experiencing some hair loss or thinning of their hair during the menopause. This may be caused by hormone imbalances (similar to the ones during pregnancy) and will usually be temporary. Equally, emotional or physical stress, illness, medication (including synthetic hormone replacement therapy [HRT]) and thyroid problems can be to blame, or hair loss at this time in life can be hereditary.

Above Enjoy your hair whatever your age. Understand changes in your body and adapt your haircare routine accordingly, and seek advice from a doctor if you are unhappy.

The thinning process often ceases after the menopause, when hormone levels have stabilized, and some women experience renewed hair growth and thickness.

Easy ways to disguise thin hair include:
▪ Have a short, layered style to add the illusion of fullness and body.
▪ Blow-dry hair in the opposite direction to growth then, when it is dry, brush it back in the other direction. This helps create root lift which makes hair appear fuller.
▪ Avoid using combs, as they will 'snag' hair and pull it out; use soft hairbrushes instead, which are kinder on the hair.
▪ Use a good volumizing mousse to add body to clean hair.
▪ Alternate the type of shampoo you use every month.

Hair colour and texture

From striking brunettes, to the lightest of blondes, fiery redheads and stunning black, colour is an important way of enhancing your look. But what makes one head of hair so different from another? Here's a quick guide to why hair varies so much.

What determines hair colour?

Hair colour is closely related to skin colour, and both are governed by the same type of pigment, melanin. The number of these melanin granules in the cortex of the hair and the shape of these granules determine a person's natural hair colour.

In the majority of cases the melanin granules are elongated in shape. People who have a large number of elongated melanin granules in the cortex of each hair have black hair, those with slightly fewer elongated granules have brown hair, and people with even less will be blonde. In other people the melanin granules are spherical or oval rather than elongated, and this makes the hair appear red.

Combinations of spherical or oval granules, perhaps with a moderate amount of the elongated ones, will give the appearance of rich, reddish-brown tinges.

If, however, spherical granules occur in combination with a large number of elongated granules, then the blackness of the hair will almost mask the redness, although it will still give a subtle tinge to the hair and differentiate it from pure black.

Below The natural colour of hair affects its texture: blonde (bottom left) is finest, brunette (below) is slightly thicker, and red hair (bottom) is thickest.

Above Asian hair tends to be black and straighter, thicker and coarser than other types.

Above Afro hair is often naturally tightly curled and dark brown in colour.

Above Caucasian hair ranges from straight to curly, and from dark brown to white blonde.

Hair colour darkens with age, but at some stage of life the pigment formation slows down. As the amount of melanin granules reduces, silvery-grey hairs begin to appear. Gradually, the production of melanin ceases and all the hair becomes colourless – which is often termed grey or white. When melanin granules are lacking from birth, as in albinos, the hair is white.

Hair texture

The natural colour of hair also affects its texture, which is determined by the diameter of each hair. Natural blondes have finer hair than brunettes, while redheads have the thickest hair. Generally speaking, hair can be divided into three categories: fine, medium, and thick and coarse, and these have certain traits:

- **Fine hair** can be strong or weak; but, because of its texture, all fine hair has the same characteristic – it lacks volume.
- **Medium hair** is neither too thick nor too thin, and is strong and elastic.
- **Thick and coarse hair** is abundant and heavy, with a tendency to grow outwards from the scalp as well as downwards. It often lacks elasticity and is frizzy.

A single head of hair may consist of several different textures. For example, fine hair is often found on the temples, and the hairline at the front and on the nape of the head, while the texture elsewhere may be medium or even coarse.

Race can determine hair texture and colour. Caucasian hair usually varies from straight to curly, while the colour ranges from dark brown to white blonde. Afro hair is usually tightly curled and dark brown, while Asian hair tends to be straight, thick, coarse and black. Mixed races will be a combination.

Did you know?

- *Healthy hair is highly elastic and can stretch 20 or 30 per cent before snapping.*
- *Chinese circus acrobats have been known to perform tricks while suspended by their hair.*
- *A human hair is stronger than copper wire of the same thickness.*
- *The combined strength of a full head of human hair is capable of supporting a weight equivalent to that of 99 people.*
- *We lose about 100 hairs a day, but as the average head has between 100,000 and 140,000 it's not a problem.*

Straight or curly?

Whether hair is curly, wavy or straight depends on two things: its shape as it grows out of the follicle; and the distribution of keratin-producing cells at the roots.

All hair grows with a twist (even when it appears to be straight) and the number of twists it takes will determine how curly it will be. For example, Afro hair has nearly 12 times as many twists as Caucasian hair.

Where the hair bulb or papilla lies in the follicle affects whether the hair grows either straighter or curlier. Where there is an even distribution of keratin cells around the bulb in the follicle, straight hair is formed. In curly hair, however, the production of keratin cells is uneven, so that at any given time there are more keratin cells on one side of the oval-shaped follicle than on the other, causing the hair to grow at an angle. In addition, the production of excess cells alternates between the sides, so the developing hair grows first in one direction and then in the other; the result is curly hair.

Define your hair type

Your hair type is determined by its natural condition – how much moisture the hair holds and its sebum levels – and how you treat your hair. Perming, colouring and heat styling can have an impact, so it is important to use the correct products.

Having established what the natural texture of your hair is, it is important to work out its type – the dryness, softness or oiliness – so that you ensure you use products that are appropriate for that type of hair.

Normal hair

This type is defined as neither oily nor dry, and has been left in its natural state. It is able to hold its style, and looks good most of the time.

Haircare Because it has not been chemically altered or damaged, normal hair may only need a conditioning treatment on an occasional basis. Choose a gentle shampoo for regular use, or you could try a two-in-one conditioning shampoo. When this dual-action product

is lathered into wet hair the shampoo removes dirt, oil and styling products while the conditioner remains in the lather. As the hair is rinsed with clean water, the oil and dirt are washed away with the shampoo and conditioning droplets are released on to the hair, leaving it shiny and easier to manage.

Dry hair

This type of hair looks dull, feels dry, tangles easily, and is difficult to comb or brush, particularly when it is wet. It simply doesn't contain enough moisture, which can be because there isn't enough sebum being produced or perhaps because the hair is older and the cuticles have opened up. When this happens, the cortex is more likely to lose its moisture through

exposure to excessive shampooing, overuse of heat-styling equipment, misuse of colour or perms, damage from the sun, or harsh weather conditions. Roughed-up cuticles mean the hair loses its ability to shine and the cortex may even split or break, making hair brittle.

Haircare Really damaged, dry hair cannot repair itself but you can help prevent further deterioration. For example, if your hair has become dry and lost its elasticity, bounce and suppleness it's important to use a nourishing shampoo and an intensive conditioner. Allowing hair to dry naturally whenever possible and reducing the amount of heat-styling from hairdryers and electrical styling tools will also help. Protect from further exposure to drying environments or UV rays.

__Below__ Hair at the roots is new and needs less conditioner, so apply to mid-lengths and ends.

__Below__ Restore bounce and vitality by using a purifying cleanser to remove product overload.

__Below__ Very curly hair may be dry and prone to breakage without moisturizing products.

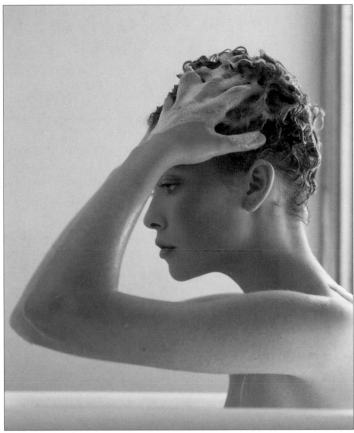

Oily hair

Often associated with teenagers, oily hair looks lank and greasy and needs frequent washing. It is caused by the overproduction of sebum, which can be a genetic tendency, or as a result of hormone disturbances, stress, a humid atmosphere, excessive brushing, constantly running hands through the hair, or perspiration, After cleansing, the hair becomes oily, sticky and unmanageable in a short time.
Haircare Use a gentle, non-aggressive shampoo that also gives the hair added volume. Consider a light perm, which will lift the hair at the roots and limit the

Did you know?

You can determine the texture of your hair by running the thumb and finger along the length of the hair from the root to the tip. Fine hair is small in diameter and feels smooth and silky along its length. Coarse hair, because of the way it is formed (a wide diameter with more raised, lifted cuticles) feels rougher to the touch. It's important to identify your hair texture in order to choose the right care and styling products.

dispersal of sebum. It could be worth rethinking your diet: reduce dairy fats and greasy foods. Try to eat plenty of fresh food, and drink six to eight glasses of water every day.

Combination hair

This common type of hair is typified by being oily at the roots but dry and sometimes split at the ends. Not only can it look lank and flat, but it will be dull and flyaway too. The causes include a reliance on chemical treatments, the overuse of detergent-based shampoos, overexposure to sunlight, and overuse of heat-styling equipment. Such repeated abuse often provokes sebum secretion at the roots and a partial alteration in the cuticle scales, which no longer protect the cortex so the hair ends become dry.
Haircare Experiment with some of the many products on offer until you find the best ones for you. Aim for those that have only a gentle action on the hair. Excessive use of formulations intended specifically for oily hair or for dry hair may contribute to the problem. Ideally, use a product

***Above left** Hair that is well cared for will be smooth and easily combed to be tangle-free.*

***Above right** Most hair is a combination of hair types so it is important to use the right products only where they are needed.*

specially designed for combination hair. If this is not possible, try using a shampoo for oily hair and finish by applying a conditioner only from the middle lengths to the ends of the hair, where moisture is needed.

Grey hair

This effect is primarily, but not always, linked with the ageing of the hair. The loss of colour is due to the gradual reduction in the amount of melanin granules produced. Grey hair is usually a mix of hair with and without colour (white hair is total loss of colour), and it tends to be coarser than younger hair.
Haircare Grey hair may absorb pollution and can even look yellow, so it's important to use products designed specifically for greying hair to give it additional protection from the environment.

Common problems

Many problems with the hair and scalp, whether naturally occurring or of our own making, can be addressed relatively easily. It's simply a question of understanding the causes and, where appropriate, taking specialist advice.

Damaged hair

Many people suffer from damaged hair, which is typified by being dull, lifeless, lacking in shine and difficult to manage. In many cases, unavoidable environmental factors, such as wind, sun, sand, sea water, chlorine, air-conditioning or central heating are the culprits, but excessive use of hairdryers and straightening or curling irons will also take their toll.

Even if you don't expose your hair to exterior stresses, the misuse of styling tools, including combs or hairbrushes, pins, hairgrips (bobby pins) and elastic hairbands (headbands) can damage the hair cuticle and make hair more brittle and appear less shiny. It is important, therefore, to be gentle with your hair at all times, even when you simply put it up in a ponytail, avoiding any ripping or tugging.

Chemical processes all work by changing the structure of hair in order to allow colour to penetrate or a perm solution to work. When perming or relaxing, the structure of the hair must be broken and then neutralized or restructured afterwards. This process means that chemically-altered hair is very often more porous than untreated hair, so it needs gentle cleansers and good conditioners.

Haircare Preventing damage is about keeping hair as flexible as possible with a high moisture content. Conditioning products are very effective; choose specific ones to address varying degrees of damage.

Limp hair

Fine hair tends to be limp, looks flat, and is difficult to handle because it does not hold a style. The texture of fine hair is hereditary, but the problem is often made worse by using too heavy a conditioner, which weighs the hair down. Excessive use of styling products can have the same effect.

Haircare To tackle the problem, wash hair frequently with a mild cleanser and use a very light conditioner. Volumizing shampoos can help give body, and soft perms will make hair appear thicker. Colouring hair can swell the hair shaft and help to add body to fine hair.

Try blow-drying hair using volumizing and styling products particularly focused on the roots, and tip your head upside-down as you direct airflow at the roots. You could also try self-grip rollers as they can help give you root lift (the longer the hair, the larger the roller should be).

Dull hair

Lacklustre hair can be caused by weathering – a combination of heat, salt, chlorine or silica build-up from the overuse of products.

Haircare Use a clarifying shampoo to deep-clean hair. Consider having ends trimmed and look for a revitalizing treatment to renourish hair and add condition and shine.

Above Be kind to your hair! Stressed hair needs special attention to recover its condition.

Static hair

Often caused by a dry atmosphere, particularly air-conditioned rooms, or hair coming into contact with synthetic materials such as nylon pillows, static is especially bad for flyaway hair, making it doubly uncontrollable.

Haircare Counter static by fixing hair in place with holding wax, gels and styling products that give the hair weight.

Frizzy hair

The merest hint of moisture being absorbed into the hair can cause frizziness. It looks dry, lacks lustre, and is difficult to control. It can also be inherited or caused by rough treatment.

Haircare To tame frizziness, massage shampoo into the roots and allow the lather to work its way to the ends. Apply a conditioner from the mid-lengths of the hair to the ends, or use a leave-in conditioner.

Alternatively, allow the hair to dry naturally and then style it using a wax or pomade. Gels with oil content and serums can also help. There are silicon-based products that work by surrounding the cuticle with a transparent microscopic film, which leaves the hair shaft smoother. Serums effectively prevent moisture loss and inhibit the absorption of dampness from the surrounding air.

Wayward curls

Messed-up curls, whether natural, on permed hair or temporarily styled, can be a pain.
Haircare Define curls more cleanly by using sculpting lotion on damp hair before setting the hair, or spritzing dry hair with curl defining spray, which gives weight and shape to tired curls.

Untrainable hair

No-hold hair which is heavy and inclined to fall out of shape.
Haircare Wayward hair can be encouraged to stay put by using a strong-hold mousse or gel spray on damp hair which is then rough-dried to about 80 per cent dry then more product applied before working that final shape. Make sure each section of hair is thoroughly dried and cooled into the required shape before moving on to the next.

Below Applying a strong-hold mousse or gel spray to damp hair before drying can help tame wayward locks.

Product build-up

This is often the residue of styling products and two-in-one shampoo formulation left on the hair shaft. When these residues combine with mineral deposits in the water, a build-up occurs, preventing thorough cleansing and conditioning. The result is dull, lacklustre, flat hair that is often difficult to perm or colour successfully because there is a barrier preventing the chemicals from penetrating the hair shaft. The colour can be patchy and the perm result uneven.
Haircare Use a stripping, chelating or clarifying shampoo, as these are specially designed to remove product build-up. This is particularly important prior to perming or colouring as it may affect the process.

Discoloured hair

Hair that is discoloured or even green can be caused by the blue dye that is used to show up the chlorine in swimming pools. Highlighted or porous hair will pick up the dye, which is absorbed into the hair shaft.
Haircare Try a detox shampoo or even concentrated tomato juice or ketchup as the red colouring neutralizes the green tinge. A hairdresser can usually help if the problem persists. Swimmers can also buy special shampoos and try wearing a swimming cap.

Below Wearing a cap when swimming will help prevent lighter hair from becoming discoloured by chlorine.

Above Although styling products are key to good-looking hair, they can result in build-up.

Misuse of hairdryers

An itchy or tight scalp may be an indication of a condition developing that needs treating, but it may simply be that you are overheating your head and causing skin to dry out and become irritated.
Haircare Try using slightly cooler water during your cleansing and conditioning routine. Hold hairdryers further away from your head (15cm/6in is ideal) and use heat-protective sprays before heat styling, as they protect the hair and the scalp from scorching. Try changing your haircare and styling products for more gentle ones. Check out new calming and soothing serums for the scalp, which are available to apply during the day or overnight. If the problem persists, seek further help.

Quick fixes for when time is short

- To revive or add volume to tired hair when there is not time to wash it, spritz the roots with blow-drying spray, then dry the hair, focusing on the roots.
- Revive naturally curly hair by spritzing with water and twisting into ringlets using your fingers.
- Wake up flat hair by tipping your head upside down and spraying the roots with hairspray – not too much or your hair will feel sticky and overloaded.
- When pinning up hair, lightly backcomb the roots to add guts and something for the pins to grip on to.

Trichoptilosis (split ends)

When hairs split at their ends it is often a sign of hair that is past its best.
Haircare The hair should be well-oiled to soften and remoisturize the dry ends. It's not possible to mend the splits – they will need to be trimmed – but applying split-end treatments may temporarily ease their unsightly appearance.

Hypertrichosis (excess hair)

This is where there is superfluous hair, or an abnormal development of hair on any area of the body where you would usually expect to find only downy hair.
Haircare This unwanted hair can be removed by tweezers or depilatory products, electrolysis, shaving or epilation, either in a salon, clinic or at home.

Trichotillomania (hair-pulling)

This is a condition when someone feels compelled to pull their hair out, usually on their scalp, perhaps in the same place, or even their eyebrows and eyelashes.
Haircare Sufferers can usually be helped through counselling, hypnosis or even drug therapies.

Alopecia (hair loss) or baldness

This is the technical term for any type of abnormal hair loss, in other words where the hair is shed and not replaced.

Diet, stress, pollution, illness and medication, and genetic factors come into play, and may have caused the hair follicle to become damaged and stop producing keratin. It may be that hormone treatments and better nutrition and mineral supplements can help slow down or halt further loss. It is also caused by medication or treatments such as chemotherapy, in which case the condition is often reversed when the treatment stops. Some of the most common types include:

▪ **Alopecia senilis** is the common form of baldness that occurs in old age. It is not permanent.
▪ **Alopecia premature** is a form of baldness that begins before middle age. The hair is shed gradually and replaced by thinner, weaker hair.

▪ **Traction alopecia** is when hair is physically stressed by being pulled back too tightly, for example into a ponytail.
▪ **Alopecia areata** is where patches of hair fall out for no apparent reason or due to injury to the nervous system. It's often associated with auto-immune disorders. Affected areas are smooth, slightly depressed and pale in colour due to decreased blood supply. Treatments and drug therapies can help. You will need to consult a doctor or trichologist.
▪ **Post-partum alopecia** occurs after having a baby and breast-feeding, when hormonal inbalances cause more hair than usual to fall out. While worrying, this usually corrects itself within months.
▪ **Alopecia totalis** is the total loss of scalp and facial hair. Hair does not normally regrow and you will need to consult a doctor or trichologist.
▪ **Alopecia universalis** is the total loss of all hair from the body and scalp. It can be caused by a major shock or an accident, and regrowth is rare. You will need to consult a doctor or trichologist.

Flaky/itchy scalp

This condition produces tiny white pieces of dead skin that flake off the scalp and are usually first noticed on the shoulders.

Below Hair loss caused by medical treatments such as chemotherapy should be temporary.

It can often be confused with dandruff but the two are not related. Sometimes the scalp is red or itchy and feels tense.

The cause could be hereditary traits, stress, insufficient rinsing of shampoo, lack of sebum, using too harsh a shampoo, vitamin imbalance, pollution, air-conditioning and central heating, and sometimes it is a side-effect of medication, including chemotherapy.
Haircare Calming serums and lotions are available (some intended to be used at night-time) and are a soothing way to tackle the problem and remoisturize the scalp. Ask a trichologist or hair salon for advice on these and on how to address the cause with improved haircare regimes and diet.

Dandruff

This happens when scaly particles with an oily sheen lie close to the hair root. The condition should not be confused with a flaky scalp, and is nothing to do with poor hygiene or stress. Causes are thought to be a microscopic fungal yeast called *Malassezia furfur*, which is present in everyone's scalp. Sometimes, when the scalp becomes irritated, skin cells produce greater amounts of the yeast, causing cells to clump together and

Below Pulling hair too tight on a regular basis can cause traction alopecia.

produce flakes of dandruff. A poor diet, sluggish metabolism, and a hormonal imbalance can make things worse. It may be that insufficient rinsing of the hair after shampooing, or the use of strong shampoos also contributes to dandruff.

Haircare Don't necessarily rush out to buy special treatment shampoos. They may be beneficial, but it's worth thinking longer term by looking at your diet and lifestyle. You could try brushing the hair before shampooing and scrupulously washing combs and hairbrushes. Always choose a mild shampoo and perhaps a moisturizing one. Avoid excessive use of heat stylers. If the dandruff persists, try specially labelled products or consult a doctor or trichologist.

Psoriasis

This condition can affect the entire scalp or just the hairline. It is typified by raised red patches covered with silvery-white scales, which can be itchy, tight and sore. It is caused by excessive skin production.

Haircare Herbal or aromatherapy products may help but it is best to consult a doctor or trichologist, who may be able to prescribe a range of treatments.

Eczema

This skin condition is typified by tight, dry and irritated skin that can become broken and sore.

Haircare It's important to use very mild cleansing products, or simply rinse hair in water if skin is irritated by soap and shampoos. Comb very gently to avoid exacerbating the problem further.

Seborrhoeic dermatitis

This is a non-infectious type of skin inflammation caused by the same fungal yeast that is responsible for dandruff. It can be aggravated by stress, or even inherited. In babies the condition is commonly called cradle cap. The tell-tale signs are large, greasy, yellowish scales that stick to the scalp; inflammation of the skin and mild patches of flaky skin on the face. In extreme cases, a rash of red, scaly skin can develop on the scalp and face.

Above Dandruff is unsightly but not something to worry about too much. Vigorous brushing before washing may help.

Haircare An anti-dandruff shampoo should help but, if not, consult a doctor or trichologist.

Sebaceous cysts

These are marble-like lumps that occur when keratin accumulates under the skin and forms single bumps or clusters of several at a time. There are not normally painful but may be big enough to catch on a hairbrush or comb.

Haircare They may need removing, so consult a doctor or trichologist.

Infection

Easily spread, infections are caused by harmful germs and bacteria. They are contagious and must be treated, and will affect the condition of the scalp and hair.
- **Bacterial infections**, such as boils and impetigo, can be treated with antibiotics. Viruses survive in all living cells of the body, so colds and flu will affect hair condition, too.
- **Fungal infections** will feed on keratin and can spread to the scalp. They include ringworm, so must be treated quickly or they may cause hair loss.

Above Regularly washing combs and brushes can help prevent problems such as dandruff, keeping your hair in superb condition.

Infestation

It's an uncomfortable fact of life that from time to time hair may become infested with lice, which transfer from head to head through direct contact. Lice often spread rapidly between children who will lean in close to each other at school or play, but equally affect adults, so it's very important to be aware of the possibility of lice transferring to other family members.

The lice lay eggs (called nits), which are very hard to dislodge. Because they need warm temperatures, the lice or nits will be found closer to the scalp rather than down the hair. They cling tenaciously to the hair shaft.

Haircare Nits and lice will literally have to be combed out using a special fine-toothed comb most commonly found at pharmacists. It's possible to buy chemical formulations, which manufacturers claim kill the lice, but their efficiency is debatable, and regular combing to both remove lice and keep further attacks at bay is highly recommended. Once the lice or nits are removed, comb the hair with a fine comb a minimum of once every three days, sterilizing the comb between uses.

Shampooing hair

Establishing an efficient and effective haircare routine starts with great cleansing. Depending on whether you are washing daily or several times a week, and on the type and needs of your hair, there are several guides you can follow.

Why shampoo?

Designed to cleanse the hair and scalp, shampoos remove dirt without stripping away too much of the natural sebum, which provides shine. They generally contain cleansing agents, perfume, preservatives and conditioning agents that can coat the hair shaft to make it appear thicker. The conditioning agents smooth the cuticle scales to help prevent the hair from tangling and eliminate static electricity from the hair when it dries.

Different types of shampoo

There is a huge range of shampoos (some of which are called cleansers or hairbaths), so it's possible to find one suited to every hair type, texture, colour or condition. It is important that you change your shampoo according to different circumstances. For example, in the summer, use a moisturizing shampoo with a sun protection factor; when colouring, use a product to help prevent colour fade; or when suffering a condition such as dandruff, opt for a specialist type.

The pH factor

This refers to the acid/alkaline level of a substance. It is calculated on a scale of 1 to 14. Numbers below 7 denote acidity, those over 7 indicate alkalinity.

Hair sebum has a pH factor of between 4.5 and 5.5, which is mildly acidic. Bacteria cannot survive in this pH, so it is important to maintain this protective layer of sebum in order to keep the skin, scalp and hair in optimum condition. If too acidic or too alkaline a product is used on hair, it may cause hair to become porous, weakened and even break.

Most shampoos range between a pH factor of 5 and 7; medicated varieties have a pH of about 7.3, which is near neutral.

Many shampoos are labelled 'pH balanced', and restore hair to its natural acidity, which is especially useful after chemical treatments such as colouring.

Scalp massage

Massage helps maintain a healthy scalp. It brings extra blood to the skin tissue, which enhances the delivery of nutrients and oxygen to the hair follicle. Massage also reduces scalp tension – which can contribute to hair loss – loosens dead skin cells, and perhaps helps redress the overproduction of sebum, which makes hair oily.

You can easily give yourself a scalp massage at home. Use warm olive oil if the scalp is dry or tight. Try equal parts of witch hazel and mineral water if you have an oily scalp. For a normal scalp, use equal parts rose and mineral waters. Simply warm the chosen ointment in your hands, apply to the scalp evenly, then

Left Once you have established a routine that suits your hair type and current condition, it can be quick and easy to maintain.

Above Just as you would alter your facial cleanser to suit your skin type, select a shampoo according to your current needs.

begin massaging your scalp at the hairline and work backwards to the base of your skull. Once you have reached the back, start again at your temples and work backwards. Use small, circular motions and medium pressure.

Tips for shampooing

- Use the correct shampoo (and not too much) for your hair type. If in doubt, use the mildest shampoo you can buy.
- Don't wash your hair in washing-up liquid, soap or other detergents; they are highly alkaline and will upset your hair's pH balance by stripping out the natural oils.
- Read the instructions for use first as every product varies slightly.
- Buy sachets of shampoo to test which brand is the most suitable for your hair.
- Never wash your hair in the bath; dirty bath water is not conducive to clean hair.
- Always wash your hairbrush and comb when you shampoo your hair.
- Don't throw away a shampoo that doesn't lather. The amount of suds is determined by the active level of detergent and some shampoos create less suds than others, but this has no effect on their cleansing ability.

Did you know?

Most of us don't spend enough time rinsing off shampoo – it really should be a step that takes at least two minutes. Avoid using water that is too hot as it may irritate and inflame the scalp.

Shampooing hair

Taking care of healthy hair starts with a great cleansing routine. It's not rocket science but there is a technique to follow that means you will maintain maximum condition for scalp and hair.

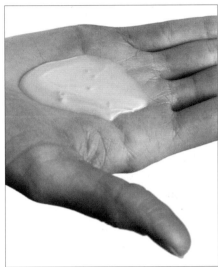

1 Wet hair thoroughly using a shower, ensuring all the layers are completely soaked through – this will activate the shampoo properly when it is applied.

2 Pour the shampoo into the palm of your hand, never directly on to the hair as it's tricky to control how much you use. For short hair you only need the same amount as a small coin, for longer hair you may require more, but never more than you can easily hold in the palm of your hand.

3 Work the shampoo through the hair, massaging your scalp and paying particular attention to the hairline around the ears and base of the neck. It should lather well but not too much.

4 Rinse away all the shampoo, then pat hair dry or squeeze gently to get rid of excess water. Don't rub or you will cause hair to tangle or break. Wet hair is more vulnerable than dry hair.

Conditioning hair

Hair in good condition is manageable, shiny, flexible and feels soft. Ideally, a simple shampoo would guarantee gorgeous results, but conditioning is often required to combat stresses caused by chemical processes, as well as to rectify problems.

Why condition?

Glossy hair has cuticle scales that lie flat and overlap, reflecting light. Perming and colouring, rough handling and heat-styling all conspire to lift the cuticles and roughen them up, both allowing moisture to be lost from the cortex and making hair dry, lacklustre, and prone to tangle. Severely damaged cuticles break off completely, leaving the hair's cortex exposed, which leads to splits and breakages.

To put the shine back into hair and restore its natural lustre it may be necessary to use a specific conditioner that meets your hair's requirements. Conditioners, with the exception of hot oils, should be applied to freshly shampooed hair that has been blotted dry with a towel so that it is damp rather than wet.

Different types of conditioners

Conditioning products are delivered in different formats and have different effects:
▪ **Basic conditioners** coat the hair with a fine film, temporarily smoothing down the cuticle and making hair glossier and easier to manage. Leave on the hair for a few minutes before rinsing thoroughly.

▪ **Leave-in conditioners**, in spray or cream format, are intended to be applied after cleansing hair. Follow the instructions on the bottle, then leave on the hair when drying and styling. They save time and are perfect for limited use when hair is extra-dry, after colouring, or when intense heat is used.

Below left Heavier masques and crème treatments can be used on a once-a-week basis to restore hair's condition.

Below Hair that is well-conditioned should feel soft, flexible and be easy to manage.

- **Conditioning sprays** are designed to be used prior to styling and form a protective barrier against the harmful effects of heat. They are also good for reducing static electricity on flyaway hair.
- **Hot oils** give an intensive, deep nourishing treatment. To use, place the unopened tube in a cup of hot tap water and leave to heat for one minute. Next, wet the hair and towel it dry before twisting off the tube top. Massage the hot oil evenly into the scalp and throughout the hair for one to three minutes. For a more intensive treatment, cover the head with a shower cap and leave to penetrate. To finish, rinse the hair, then shampoo.
- **Intensive conditioning treatments** can be applied both in a salon – often as part of a ritual or service – or for occasional use at home. They may be rich crèmes or masques, and using them will help hair to retain its natural moisture balance, replenishing it where necessary. Use particularly if the hair is split, dry, frizzy, or difficult to manage.
- **Restructurants** penetrate the cortex, helping to repair and strengthen the inner part of damaged hair. They are helpful if the hair is lank and limp and has lost its natural elasticity as a result of chemical treatments or physical damage.
- **Split-end treatments and serums** condition damaged hair. The best course of action for split ends is to have the ends trimmed, but this does not always solve the whole problem because the hair tends to break off and split at different levels. As an intermediate solution, split ends can appear to be temporarily sealed using these specialist conditioners.
- **Colour/perm conditioners** are designed for chemically-treated hair. After-colour products add a protective film around porous areas of the hair, preventing colour loss. After-perm products help stabilize the hair, thus keeping the bounce in the curl.

Did you know?

If you find your hair becomes oilier more quickly than usual, it may be that your conditioner is too heavy. Don't immediately discard it, rather try rinsing if off sooner than usual, and perhaps applying less.

Conditioning hair

Most hair that has been treated with a chemical process or exposed to environmental stresses will need either regular or occasional conditioning treatments after shampooing. Be careful not to apply too much conditioner – a little is designed to go a long way, and using too much product will make the hair feel lank and weighed down.

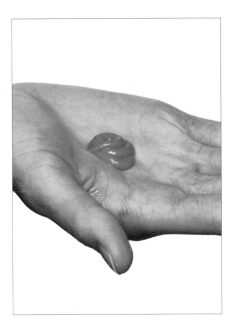

1 Follow the instructions on the packaging, but as a general guide, use only a large coin-sized amount of product on mid-length hair, and less on shorter hair.

2 Rub the product lightly over the palms of both hands to make it easier to apply, then distribute it evenly along the lengths of damp (not soaking wet), cleansed hair.

3 Work the product through the mid-lengths and ends rather than trying to massage it into the scalp, which is not usually necessary since the root area is new growth, which should be in a good condition naturally. Comb through hair gently using a wide-tooth comb to ensure the conditioner is evenly distributed. This type of comb is less likely to pull and break hair than other smaller-toothed combs. The conditioner should make it easy to detangle the hair. Wait the indicated amount of time (usually 2–5 minutes) to allow the conditioner to penetrate, before rinsing off with warm water. Towel dry, then comb again.

Natural treatments

In cultures the world over, herbs and plants have been used to heal and beautify. Many of these age-old haircare recipes are still useful today and you may find them worth a try. Use them immediately after you have made them; they won't keep.

Herbal shampoo

Crush a few dried bay leaves with a rolling pin and mix with a handful of dried camomile flowers and one handful of rosemary. Place in a large jug and pour over 1 litre/1¾ pints/4 cups boiling water. Strain after 2–3 minutes and mix in 5ml/1 tsp of soft or liquid soap. Apply to the hair, massaging well for a minute or two. Rinse thoroughly.

For condition and shine:

- **Egg mask** Blend two eggs with 30ml/ 2 tbsp water and 15ml/1 tbsp cider vinegar or lemon juice. Massage into damp hair and leave for 10–15 minutes before rinsing thoroughly with lukewarm (not hot) water.
- **Banana mask** Mix together 1 mashed banana, 45ml/3 tbsp honey, 45ml/3 tbsp milk, 75ml/5 tbsp olive oil and 1 egg. Apply to damp hair and massage so it is evenly distributed. Leave on the hair for up to 30 minutes, then rinse thoroughly and shampoo and condition your hair as usual.

- **Yogurt mask** Prepare by blending 105ml/7 tbsp plain (natural) yogurt with the beaten white of 1 egg. Apply to damp hair, massage through the roots to ends and leave for up to 30 minutes. Shampoo and condition your hair as usual.
- **Avocado, honey and olive oil** are also great hair conditioners. You can use them in different combinations (olive oil whisked with egg, or honey and olive oil blended in equal parts) or all together. Simply conjure up a consistency to suit you, leave on as long as you like to work their magic, and then shampoo and rinse hair well.

Rinses (after shampooing)

Lemon juice added to the rinsing water will brighten blonde hair, while 30ml/2 tbsp of cider vinegar will add gloss and body to any colour hair.

Other rinses (to be used after shampooing) can be made up to treat a variety of problems. First you must make an infusion by placing 30ml/2 tbsp of a fresh herb in a china or glass bowl. Fresh herbs are best, but if you are using dried

Left Banana and avocado fruit make nourishing hair masks.

ones, remember they are stronger so you will need to halve the amount required for fresh herbs. Add 600ml/1 pint boiling water, cover and leave to steep for three hours. Strain before using. Try:

- **Southernwood** to combat oiliness.
- **Nettle** to stimulate hair growth.
- **Rosemary** to prevent static.
- **Lavender** to soothe a tight scalp.
- **Tea tree** to ward off infestation.

Using essential oils

Pure aromatherapy oils can be used for hair care. The following recipes come from world-famous aromatherapist Robert Tisserand. The number of drops of oil, as listed, should be diluted in 30ml/ 2 tbsp (or two large spoons) of vegetable oil, which will act as a carrier oil:

- **Dry hair**: rosewood 9, sandalwood 6.
- **Oily hair**: bergamot 9, lavender 6.
- **Dandruff**: eucalyptus 9, rosemary 6.

Mix the required treatment and apply to dry or wet hair. Massage the scalp using the fingertips. Leave for 2–5 minutes. Shampoo and rinse thoroughly.

Left Let natural essential oils work their magic, restoring hair condition, shine and vitality and combating dandruff.

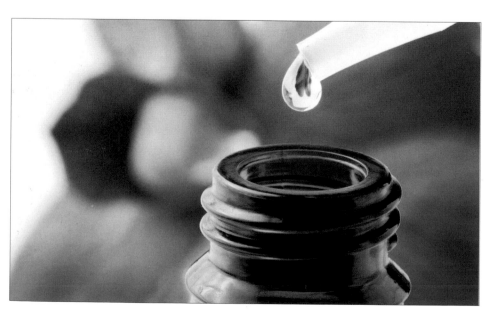

Happy holidays

More damage can be done to hair during a two-week holiday in the sun than over the rest of the year! To ensure your hair enjoys the break as much as you do, it is important that you prepare well and pack products to keep you looking perfect all holiday long.

Almost every aspect of a holiday in the sun can wreak havoc on our hair. The ultraviolet rays or radiation (UVRs) from sunlight that can cause damage to the skin also have an adverse affect on hair, depleting it of natural oils and removing moisture. White hair is particularly susceptible to the effects of the sun because it has lost its natural pigmentation (melanin), which would normally help to filter out harmful UVRs to a certain extent.

Exposure to strong winds can whip treated hair into a tangle, causing breakage and split ends, while chlorinated and salt water cause colour to fade and treated hair to weaken and dry out substantially faster than untreated hair. As if that wasn't bad enough, chlorine can also cause blonde, grey or white hair to take on a greenish tinge.

Sun and wind protection

Protecting your hair as well as your skin from the sun's harmful rays makes sense. This can be done by wearing a hat or a scarf and using a specially formulated product. Sunscreen sprays and gels are available for the hair and these offer a good deal of protection. Comb them through your hair and leave on all day.

Remember to reapply the product after swimming. Alternatively, use a leave-in conditioner, choosing one that protects the hair against UVRs.

On windy or blustery days, keep long hair tied back to prevent tangles. Long hair can also be plaited (braided) when it is wet and the plait left in all day, which offers some protection. When evening comes and you undo the plaits, you will have a cascade of rippling curls.

Below Be kind to your hair and make sure your two-week holiday isn't going to leave you with problem hair for the rest of the season.

If your hair does get tangled by the wind, untangle it gently using a wide-tooth comb to reduce risk of tearing and snagging, and spritz hair with conditioning spray to ease the combing process.

Holiday care

You may want to wash your hair more often than normal while on holiday. Generally speaking, you should always wash it at least once a day if you have been in a swimming pool or on the beach to get rid of salt, chlorine and sand build-up. This is perfectly fine and, contrary to the popular myth, won't mean that your hair becomes oilier and requires more washing on your return home. Even if you don't shampoo hair every time, always rinse the salt or chlorinated water thoroughly from hair after a swim, using plenty of fresh, clean water. If there is no shower, fill an empty bottle with tap water and use that instead.

Natural highlights

Exposure to the sun will fade your hair colour and make it appear lightened, which many people like. But remember this is a drying action, so you will need to replace lost moisture with conditioner. Too much sun can also burn the scalp. Applying lemon juice to speed up the lightening process is not advised, as not only is there debate over its effectiveness, but the natural citric acid can be damaging.

Pre-trip action

▪ Any hair colouring you are planning should be done at least one week prior to your holiday. This will allow time for the colour to 'soften' and for you to apply intensive conditioning on any dry ends.
▪ If you want to have a perm, book the appointment at least three weeks before departure to allow hair to settle and for you to learn how to manage your new style.

Above right It is vital that you wash, or at least rinse your hair after swimming in the sea or in a swimming pool.

Right A sun hat and a few sun-protection products, including a bottle of water, are must-haves for trips to the beach.

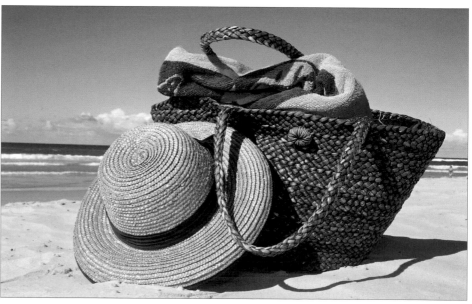

- Have your hair trimmed before you go, but do not try a radical style as you won't want to worry about coping with a new look. Whatever you do, don't have your hair cut abroad. Wait until you are back home and can visit your regular stylist.

On the beach

Exposed to sun, sand, and salt or chlorinated water, your hair will require a little extra care. Here are a few top tips:

- Tie hair at the nape of the neck rather then piling it on top of your head. This protects the ends from over-exposure to the sun.
- Take a bottle of tap water to the beach so you can rinse salt water out of your hair during the day.
- Reapply hair protection during the day as often as you would body protection. One spritz in the morning is not enough.
- Use covered hairbands (headbands) to tie back hair. Keep a scarf handy to tie hair back and cover it up in emergencies.
- In small quantities, you can use skin-protection body lotions or sprays on the hair and scalp.

On the piste

Although we may not realize it, cold temperatures, wind and reflected winter sunlight can be just as damaging to hair as beach conditions. It is important to follow these basic rules:

- The sun's rays are intensified by being reflected by snow, so hair needs extra protection in the form of a hair sunscreen.
- Wind, blasts of snow, and bright sunshine are a damaging combination for hair, so wear a hat whenever possible.
- In freezing temperatures hair picks up static electricity, making it flyaway and unmanageable. Calm the static by spraying your hairbrush with hairspray before brushing your hair.
- With sudden temperature changes and constantly changing headgear, your hair may need daily shampooing. Use a mild shampoo and light conditioner.

Right A hat is the best way to protect hair from environmental stresses, such as cold and glare from the sun bouncing off snow.

Back home

Your holiday is over, but while a tan fades quickly, the negative effects it has had on your hair may be noticeable for some time to come. Here are some easy ways to combat the more common problems:

- Use a clarifying shampoo or treatment to remove deep deposits of dirt and build-up of holiday styling products. Remember to stop using it, however, once hair is back in condition.
- Dry or flaky scalp often occurs due to over-exposure to sun, sand and wind. Applying an intensive deep-conditioning treatment that includes a scalp treatment to rehydrate the skin will help.

- Book in for a trim to get rid of over-dry or split ends.
- When on holiday it's tempting to over-indulge in a little too much food and wine, and your diet may vary quite a bit from what your body is used to. Just like your skin, your hair will be affected, so once home, calm things down with a detox diet!
- If you have acquired a greenish tinge (lightened hair is most at risk), then a detoxifying shampoo should help. Or, try applying concentrated tomato juice or ketchup to the hair as the red colouring should neutralize any green. If it won't budge, then visit the salon for a specialist deep-cleanse treatment.

Pack a bag

With the luxury of a large bathroom cabinet to store all the products you need to create different looks, it can be a headache deciding what to pack when you have to travel. Here are few ideas on what should be included depending on what size bag you have.

When planning a trip, you need to consider how long you are going for, what you will be doing and how much space you have in your luggage. Think through what activities and appointments you have and how you might want to style your hair. Do you need styling lotions, mousse, serums and spray? All will be available in travel sizes or you can decant them into smaller containers.

Go large
If room isn't a major factor but weight is, then just include the following products and equipment:
- Appropriate-sized bottles and tubs of your favourite shampoo and conditioner.
- Moisturizing conditioning treatment for use once or twice a week on a long trip. You can opt for vials or sachets rather than a large pot when you only plan to use a small amount.

Right *You can buy miniature versions of many hair-styling products, or buy small, empty containers and fill them yourself.*

- Detox shampoo to combat a change of environment, including heat, dust, or smog.
- Dry shampoo for whenever you don't have time to follow your normal routine.
- Nearly finished canisters of mousse, spray and gel are great for travel as you can use them up and discard them.
- Covered hairbands (headbands) or hair slides (barrettes) are ideal for tying hair back, whatever the occasion.
- Combs, including a wide-tooth comb.
- A large, round brush for smooth, sleek styling or creating flicks and curl.
- If possible, take a travel hairdryer with dual voltage.
- Pack an adaptor plug suitable for the country you are visiting.
- If you're travelling to somewhere hotter or colder than you are used to, take a scarf and a hat for ultimate protection. Sun hats in cotton can be folded small and woolly ski hats are a fun style statement.
- Battery or gas-powered stylers are now widely available in a range of sizes and are convenient for holidays, but remember they must be carried in the hold of the aircraft, not in your hand luggage. Refill cylinders are not allowed on aeroplanes, so make sure you fit a new cartridge before you go.
- Soft, bendy rods or self-grip rollers are a good alternative to heated ones – they are also kinder to the hair.

Medium size
If you need to travel a little lighter, then here are some easy ideas for condensing the essentials:
- Sachets of products – shampoo and conditioner, styling lotion – are perfect for travelling. Not only do they squash flat with no fear of leaking, but you can discard them as you go.
- A small tub of talcum powder can double as dry shampoo.
- Hairbands (headbands) and hairgrips (bobby pins) are small, very useful and easy to pack.
- Combs, including a wide-tooth comb, are always required.
- It is worth calling where you are staying to check if a hairdryer will be supplied.
- Mini straightening irons (even handbag irons are available) not only heat quickly but take little room. You can pep up fringes and flicks in no time.
- Self-grip rollers are bulky but light and can prove valuable if your hair goes limp.
- A scarf can protect hair and be a stylish accessory for a range of occasions. A silk scarf can also be wrapped around hair at night to reduce static if hotel pillows and air-conditioning are creating static and frizz.

Left A good way to disguise oily hair when you don't have time to wash it and don't have dry shampoo is apply talcum powder on to the roots, then brush it out.

Must-haves

Although you can get by without many products, most hair types do require a few basic help-out items:

- **Coloured hair** can fade in sunlight, so pack products to prevent or limit colour fade and keep you looking fabulous. Cold weather and wind can be very drying and make hair brittle, so keep your hair well-conditioned.
- **Fine hair** requires a gentle daily shampoo and a light, leave-in conditioner. Hairsprays are also needed to hold down the cuticle of the hair and keep out moisture in humid conditions and reduce static in cold environments.
- **Curly hair** needs a gentle moisturizing shampoo and creamy conditioner to guard against dryness from sun or air-conditioning, plus a deep-conditioning treatment for occasional use.
- **Frizzy hair** benefits from a sun- or heat-protection spray or oil, a hair mask for intensive treatment if the hair becomes too dry, and a good anti-frizz serum to calm hair and lock in moisture whatever the weather.

Double-ups

Sometimes, despite the best planning, you may forget something. There's often no need rush out to buy a replacement, however, simply see if you can use one of our clever subsitutes instead:

- **No dry shampoo?** Tip talcum powder on to the roots of your hair where it will absorb any excess oil, then brush it out thoroughly. Dabbing witch hazel on to roots will also absorb any oil. Both these techniques will work for one day, but you will then need to shampoo your hair properly.

Left and above Lightweight rollers and covered hairbands (headbands) are an essential part of a savvy stylist's washbag.

Travelling light

When you are very short of space or only going away for couple of nights, it's possible to create a neat haircare kit that contains all the vitals for cool styles:

- Two-in-one shampoo and conditioners are available in small travel sizes or sachets, which you can discard as you go. In the short-term, it's fine to use them on a daily basis. (After prolonged use they can cause product build-up, so only use them for a few days.)
- A small bottle or tube of serum multi-tasks as a quick way to calm flyaways, smooth out frizz and add instant shine.
- Take a miniature styling spray, which can be used for hold, to pep-up tired hair by spritzing the roots, or as a protector against heat- and wind-stress.
- Take enough matt hairgrips (bobby pins) to fix a chignon or up-do, both of which are great ways of dealing with 'day-old' hair. Matt rather than shiny ones won't show so much and will grip better.
- Covered hairbands (headbands) are invaluable – when all else fails, tie your hair back!
- Always include a hairbrush and/or comb.

Above When space is limited, rationalizing the contents of your washbag will mean you are never less than prepared!

- **No conditioner?** See if you can get an avocado, some honey or some oil! Blend the ingredients (mashing up the avocado) and work the mixture into damp, clean hair. Leave it to penetrate for a few minutes, then shampoo and rinse off thoroughly.
- **No serum?** Leave-in conditioner can be applied to the ends of the hair like serum to smooth and remoisturize dry ends. Hairspray will also calm flyaways and reduce frizz.
- **No heat-protector spray?** Sun-protection body lotions and oils can be applied to the hair (don't use too much) to protect your scalp and hair from the sun. Make sure they have a suitable sun protection factor (SPF).
- **No rollers?** Firm-hold mousse can be used to create curl. Apply all over damp hair, then take small sections and twist them from roots to ends. Dry slowly using a diffuser attachment on the hairdryer or leave hair to dry naturally.
- **No tongs?** Braid damp hair and leave it to dry for as long as possible – overnight if you want – to create waves and gentle curl. The tighter the braid, the tighter the curl.
- **No accessories or ornaments?** Use jewellery to add a little fun to holiday hair. Drape lightweight bracelets or charms into the hair and secure the ends with hairgrips (bobby pins), or use a brooch to double as a hair ornament.

Successful styling

Choosing a hairstyle that suits your looks and your lifestyle means considering several factors, from the cut and styling it involves to the colour and chemical treatments that may be needed. Having achieved the perfect style, you also need to learn how to maintain it and ensure a fabulous finish every time. Today, there are many styling products and tools to help, but so much choice can be overwhelming. The trick is not only to figure out what to use and when, but how they work for you in particular, given your hair type and texture. Follow our guide and have fun!

New style, new you

Looking for a new style? Fantastic. A fresh cut, colour or restyle is a great way to revamp your look and boost your confidence. However, it is important that you put some thought into what you want to achieve before you arrive at the salon.

For many women, a dramatic change – such as going from long to short, straight to curly, or brunette to blonde – coincides with a big life change, perhaps the end of a relationship or new job. It's a form of liberation and can be a great springboard into a dynamic new attitude. But be wary of making drastic decisions if you are less than 100 per cent certain. Your bravado today could be your misery tomorrow, as many changes take months to grow out and are not easily reversed.

If there's any chance you might regret your actions then go for a change with fewer commitments, such as restyling hair to include a fringe (bangs) or opting to lift or darken hair colour several tones rather than going for a complete change.

A look for a lifestyle

When browsing the pictures in this book and in magazines, think about which looks suit your age and stage. A trend can be adopted completely, or your hairdresser can incorporate an aspect of a popular look into a style – maybe a fringe detail, a colour, or texture.

Think about how much time you are prepared to spend on styling each day and whether you have the capability to maintain an elaborate look yourself. If you play sports or swim, then will daily washing and restyling require more time than you have to spare? Being a busy mum or working away a lot could also make some looks too high maintenance for your lifestyle.

Above left It is well worth flicking through fashion magazines and the galleries in this book to help you decide what style you want.

Left Lifestyle activities may dictate how long or short your hair needs to be. If you do a lot of sport, you will need to wear it tied back.

Caution pays

There are a few imaginative ways to try out a new look before you sign up for the real deal. Wanting to go from long to short? Pop on a wig or two to see how it feels. Similarly, if you want a dramatically different new colour, try a temporary hair piece in the new hue to see how it suits. A perm can be 'tried out' by getting your hair wrapped in heated rollers or bendie rods for a practice run. A good hair salon will be able to advise you not only on how a cut might suit you, but also how different hair colours will look against your skin tone.

Versatility

Talk to your hairdresser about different ways you will (or won't) be able to style your new look to suit your lifestyle, both at work and play. Will you still be able to draw hair into a ponytail for going to the gym? Can you style a new short look to be smooth or textured? How will you wear this new look for smart daytime events, or glamorous evenings out?

Thinking ahead

It's important to plan where this new hairstyle will take you. If you fancy having a short crop, then consider how long it will take to grow out and what styles you might prefer in the future. It could make sense to go for a short one-length bob that grows out quite quickly rather than a close-cut, gamine style that will take longer to move into something else.

What about colour? Adopting a new block colour will mean regrowth coming through more obviously – so consider if you have the budget to continue having roots touched up, or whether highlights are a more practical way for you to change colour without breaking the bank.

If you really want a new look that requires more hair length or volume than you currently have, then discuss with your hairdresser ways that you can work towards achieving that look in a few months time. If you hanker after one-length hair, or hate your fringe, then growing out steep layers can take up to 12 months, but it's possible to have styles and cuts in the meantime that won't compromise your end goal.

Above Consider how versatile a new look will be – taking you from day to night, for example.

When looking for a new style remember to consider:
- Why are you doing it? Is this really something you want to commit to?
- Do you have the right texture, volume and length of hair to achieve your desired style? In-salon consultations are free and talking with a hairdresser will give you a realistic perspective on what is possible for your hair and what could suit you best.
- Are you going to need a new wardrobe to complement a new colour, or hair length?
- How much styling time will your new look require and are you prepared to invest?
- Get inspiration from looking at others around you, friends, magazines and celebrities. Remember, however, to think about how that style will look on you; don't be dazzled solely by how it looks on them.
- Where will this new style take you? If you've spent the past couple of years trying to grow out a fringe, then will this new style put you right back where you started, or is it halfway to the next look?

Choosing a style

When it comes to choosing the perfect style, there are plenty of easy-to-follow guidelines on what cut best suits which face-shape, hair texture and type. But for all the advice, really the only rule is that you must feel confident and happy in yourself.

Fashions come and go with different trends and ideas, but essentially, if you learn to make the most of your looks by choosing a style that maximizes your best features, you will exude vitality and vigour and look beautiful because of it.

Face shapes

Understanding your face shape will help get you started. Is your face round, oval, square, heart-shaped or long? By defining your face shape and working with your stylist on a cut and style, you can minimize or emphasize different aspects of a face. Effects could include opening up the face and making the best of small eyes, revealing a great eyebrow shape, softening a strong jaw-line or giving the illusion of shortening a long chin.

If you are not sure what shape your face is, then the easiest way to find out is to draw the hair back off your face. Stand squarely in front of a mirror and use a lipstick to trace the outline of your face on to the mirror. When you stand back you should be able to see into which of the following categories your face shape falls: square, round, oval, heart-shaped or oblong.

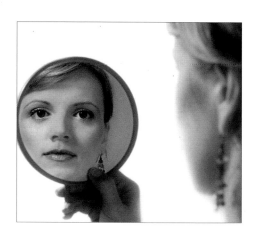

Above *Take time to consider your face shape and which features you want to emphasize.*

The square face is angular with a broad forehead and a square jawline. To make the best of this shape, choose a hairstyle with long layers, preferably one with gentle waves or curls, as these create a softness that detracts from the hard lines. Consider off-centre partings, loose curls and graduated cuts. Avoid blunt fringes (bangs).

On the round face, the distance between the forehead and the chin is about equal to the distance between the cheeks. Look at feathered haircuts where the hair falls forward to slim down a fuller face. A short fringe (bangs) will seem to lengthen the face, while a shorter cut can be more flattering than a long style.

The oval face has wide cheekbones that taper down into a small, often pointed, chin, and up to a fairly narrow forehead. This is regarded by many experts as the perfect face shape, which looks good with almost any style. Now consider your facial features – do you prefer to emphasize your mouth, eyes, cheekbones or nose?

Left A good hairstyle should match your clothes style and suit your body shape.

The complete you

When choosing a new style you should also take into account your overall body shape and your personal lifestyle. If you are a traditional pear-shape, perhaps don't go for neat, elfin styles as they accentuate a small head shape and allow attention to be drawn to the lower half of your body, making your hips look even wider. Petite women might avoid styles with masses of very curly hair as this makes the head appear larger and out of proportion with the body.

If you wear glasses, try to choose frames and a hairstyle that complement each other. Large spectacles could spoil the look of a neat, feathery cut, while very fine frames could be overpowered by a large, voluminous style. Remember to take your glasses to the salon when having your hair restyled, so that your stylist can take their shape into consideration when helping you decide on a cut.

To minimize signs of ageing, opt for a neater, more sophisticated cut, which can knock years off your look – leaving more tousled, casual styles to younger women. Don't get stuck in a style rut. Nothing is more dating than a tired look. Re-energize yourself with a new style from time to time. It doesn't have to be drastic, but a variation on a cut or colour works wonders for your appearance and for your mood.

Feature notes

You can use hairstyles to help disguise features that you don't particularly like:
- **Prominent nose?** Incorporate softness into your style.
- **Pointed chin?** Style the hair with width at the jawline.
- **Low forehead?** Choose a style with a wispy fringe (bangs), rather than one with a full fringe.
- **High forehead?** Disguise a large forehead with a full fringe.
- **Receding chin?** Select a style that comes just below chin level, with waves or curls.
- **Uneven hairline?** A fringe should help conceal this problem.

The heart-shaped face, where the widest point is at eye-level and then it tapers down to a neater chin shape, can be balanced by creating volume or width at chin level. A bob that flicks out just below the ears for example, can look fabulous. Or create volume at chin level with curls, layers or shattered perimeters.

The oblong face is characterized by a high forehead and long chin, and needs a haircut that gives the illusion of width to balance it. Soften the effect with short layers, or go for a bob with a fringe (bangs), which will create horizontal lines. Scrunch-dried or curly bobs balance a long face, too.

Choosing a hairdresser

A fantastic haircut, an eye-catching new style and gorgeous hair that is well groomed and exudes health and vitality all play a major part in how we feel, so it's important to find a hairdresser you trust to care for, cut and colour your hair.

Going to the hairdresser can be expensive, and the outcome is likely to last for a few weeks, so it's worth really taking the time to find one that suits you.

Understand your hairdresser

Hairdressers are trained to care for hair and learn how to cut, colour, style and treat it. They should also be practised in assessing which looks are best suited to which face shapes, how to assess hair types and textures, and which colours will or won't work well with different skin tones and complexions. Add to this their ability to interpret fashion trends and pass on knowledge about new products and services, and a good hairdresser is worth their weight in gold.

Before any hair appointment, you should expect a consultation with your hairdresser. The purpose of this is for them to find out what you want and to decide on a safe, appropriate and effective service to ensure you get the perfect result.

Choose a salon

Word of mouth is often the best way to select a new salon. Ask around, particularly friends or acquaintances whose hair you admire (they'll be flattered). Think about practicalities: How you will get to the salon? Is there parking?; Are their appointment times likely to suit? Do they open at weekends or have a late night? Remember that the exterior of a salon can be deceptive, so have a look at the interior as well. Go in for a chat with one of the stylists – don't be shy as salons expect this to happen and should be happy to help.

Right A visit to the salon should be a relaxing and enjoyable experience, so don't put up with service that's not perfect.

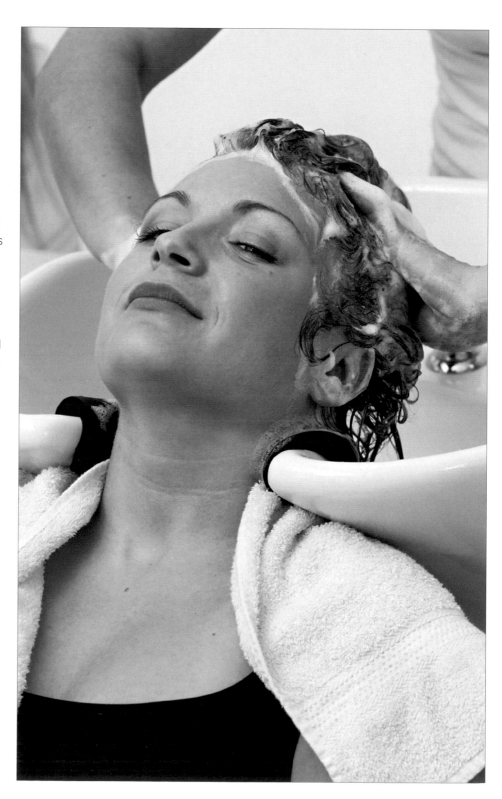

What makes a good salon

The best hairdressers look after you from the moment you call to book, right through to when you leave. These days you should expect a good level of customer service as well as high standards in hairdressing itself. The salon should have regard for your comfort and safety, especially when using chemical processes such as colouring and perming solutions. Cleanliness should also be a priority – including the personal hygiene of the stylists.

What's a good haircut?

One you can maintain at home! It's really as simple as that. If you are as happy with your hair a week later as on the day you left the salon, then it's a good sign.

How to get good advice

Build up a rapport with your hairdresser. They are not mind-readers, so try to communicate well with them so that they can offer good advice. Show them pictures of styles you like on other people (you could take in this book and show them one of the looks in the gallery section), or photographs of looks you've enjoyed wearing in the past. Talk with them about your lifestyle and how much time you are willing to spend on your hair each day. It's no good asking for a high-maintenance look if you've not got time to devote to styling before you get going each day.

At every salon visit be interested in the products used on your hair – professional products are usually high-performance but cost more too, so make sure you understand how to get the best out of them. Be clear and honest about your haircare regimes and share any concerns you have about the condition of your hair and scalp.

How to get good service

It will help set things off on the right foot if you follow these simple guidelines:
- Turn up on time.
- Be fair.
- Give feedback.
- Take advice.
- If you have to cancel, give notice.
- Don't rush your stylist.

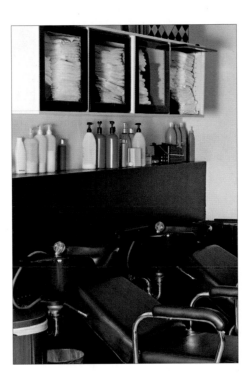

Above Most salons pride themselves on being places where you can feel pampered, paying great attention to detail, including comfort.

How to complain

It's important to speak up if you're not happy with a visit to the salon for whatever reason. The hairdresser or salon owner has a business to run, which relies not only on your custom but on satisfied customers' recommendations, so they should be grateful for the opportunity to put matters right and to be made aware of any problems.

To get the best results be clear about what it is that isn't right – is it the cut or colour, the service, treatment or price that bothers you? When you make the complaint at the salon, remember:
- Keep calm.
- Ask to see the salon manager.
- Set out what it is that you expected (in terms of hairstyle, service or price).
- Explain what it is that is different from what you expected.

If you realize that you're still not happy after you've left the salon then call the salon as soon as possible and ask to speak to the manager again. Explain once more what your expectations are and how they've not been met.

Above It takes effort from both client and stylist to build up a good rapport and is certainly worth the effort.

If your hair has been badly permed, don't accept any offer to have it re-permed, as this could exacerbate the problem. The remedy is to have a course of intensive conditioning treatments, which the salon may offer for free. Following this, you should wait until the hair is in optimum condition before you have another perm or colour treatment – this can unfortunately take a long time if you have long hair and you may want to consider having your hair shortened to remove some of the damaged hair and speed the recovery process.

If you feel you have suffered serious damage, for example an itchy, burning scalp, blisters, cuts, hair breakage or hair loss, then immediately seek advice from your family doctor or a trichologist. If they feel that you have cause for complaint and compensation, then ask them to prepare a report giving full details and an analysis of the problem. However, remember that hair grows, blisters heal, and memories fade, so act quickly and, if necessary, make sure you have some photographs taken at the time to reinforce your claim.

Cutting hair

Cutting hair properly is a skill that requires great expertise. To create a desired shape, it's important to know where weight and bulk needs to be removed to achieve a good line and balance, emphasize good points and detract from bad ones.

Hair growth varies over different parts of the head, which means that your cut can appear out of shape very quickly. As a general rule, a short, precision cut needs trimming every four weeks; a longer style every six to eight weeks. If you want to grow your hair long, it is essential to have it trimmed regularly – at least every three months – to prevent splitting and to keep the ends even. There are different ways to cut hair and even if you don't do it yourself, it's a good idea to have some understanding of techniques to help communicate more effectively with your hairdresser.

Classic cuts

Hairdressers learn the fundamental classic cuts, all of which can have variations to achieve different end results:
- **The one-length bob** is also known as a pageboy. It's a haircut where the hair falls to a one-length point that is the same all the way round the head (the perimeter) and usually sits above the shoulders. It's a useful way of making fine hair look thicker and more dense.

Variations on a classic bob cut can then be used to individualize the look, such as making the front lengths longer than the back or vice versa. The hair is cut to form a smooth edge so that the lengths gradually rise or fall around the perimeter.

The bob can be cut with or without a fringe (bangs) and with a central or side-parting. The hair can be blow-dried around a hairbrush to curl out or under, or combed to hang straight.
- **A long one-length cut** is where hair falls to a point below the shoulders. Again it can be personalized with or without a fringe and be blow-dried square-shaped or more rounded.
- **Layers** are where horizontal sections of hair are cut to the same length all round the head, so that in effect the haircut mirrors the head shape with top layers falling to a higher point than lower layers. It is useful for thinning out thick hair and removing bulk. You can have layers any length, from short to long,
- **Graduation** is a technique used to create top layers which are shorter than underneath layers. You can create a greater or lesser degree of graduation or create reverse graduation where underneath layers are shorter than top layers. It's an important technique for shaping styles.
- **A square-layered cut** is sometimes called box layers or graduated layers, and combines layering and graduation. It's called a square layer because if all the hair were blown back off the face it would form a square shape.
- **A round layered cut**, also called a French crop, is a basic layered shape where the hair is cut into rounded layers, creating a softer end shape.

Clockwise, from top left Graduated cut with a fringe; long bob with a fringe; layered hair with a short fringe; long one-length hair.

Above Angling scissors will cut either blunt lines or chip into the ends of the hair, creating different finished effects.

Cutting techniques

Ways of cutting hair vary according to the effect you want to achieve, but there are several basic techniques that a hairdresser is likely to use:

- **Blunt cutting** is when the ends of the hair are cut straight across – often used for hair of one length or definite lines.
- **Point cutting** is where the scissors are pointed into the haircut to break up straight lines and add texture.
- **Slide cutting** is a way to thin thick hair and give a soft finish. This technique is often done when the hair is dry using open scissors to slice the hair.
- **Razor cutting** is literally using a razor rather than scissors, and creates softness, tapering, and internal movement so that the hair moves freely. It can also be used to shorten hair.
- **Thinning** is done either with thinning scissors or a razor; it removes bulk and weight without affecting the overall length of the hair.

Clever cuts

The art of hairdressing is in applying different techniques and cuts to make the most of a client's hair type and texture. These are some of the most common tricks of the trade:

- Fine, thin, flyaway hair can be given volume and movement by blunt cutting.
- Mid-length hair can benefit from being lightly layered to give extra volume.
- Short, thin hair can be blunt cut and the edges graduated to give movement.
- Some hairdressers razor-cut fine hair to give a thicker and more voluminous effect. It is best not to let fine hair grow too long. As soon as it reaches the shoulders it tends to look wispy.
- Thick and coarse hair can be controlled by reducing the weight to give more style. Avoid very short styles because the hair will stick out. Try a layered cut with movement.

Did you know?

Most salons offer the chance to return between appointments to request a fringe (bangs) be trimmed at no charge. It may be that you are expected to book, depending on how busy they are.

Top A widow's peak can look very attractive if the hair is cut in a suitable style.

Above Cowlicks can be difficult to style or tame, so it is important that the hairdresser thinks carefully about how to cut the hair.

- Layering also helps achieve height and eliminates weight. On shorter styles, the weight can be reduced with thinning scissors expertly used on the ends only.

Styling problems

Sometimes hair grows in different directions, which may cause styling problems.

- **A cowlick** is found on the front hairline and occurs when the hair grows in a swirl, backwards and then forwards. Clever cutting can redistribute the weight and go some way to solving this problem.
- **A double crown** occurs when there are two pivots of natural hair at the top of the head, rather than the usual one. Styles with height at the crown are most suitable.
- **A widow's peak** is a descending point on the hairline, forming a V-shape, usually above the forehead. Taking hair in the reverse direction to the growth will give the impression of a natural wave.

Colouring hair

Beautiful hair is about condition and colour. You may be blessed with fantastic natural colour but still fancy a change, or maybe your own colouring needs a boost. Perhaps you like to change your hair tone as often as your clothes. The good news is, you can!

Technological advances in the past few years mean that hair colorants have never been better, both in terms of product efficiency and colour choice. You can now choose between temporary, semi-permanent, demi-permanent and permanent colour, Each offers a different lasting power depending on the base or natural colour, of your hair.

Different shades

Professional hair colours are made up of codes which follow an international numbering system. The first number refers to your natural hair colour, or base, and is counted from 0 (a natural blue/black) to 9 (extra light blonde). After a point, a second number indicates the tone of the hair. For instance, .0 is matt while .7 is violet. A third number indicates a secondary tone. So 6 will be Dark Blonde, while 6.4 indicates Dark Copper Blonde and 6.46 denotes Dark Copper Red Blonde.

It's not necessary to learn the numbering system but it can be useful to ask your hairdresser which numbers they have applied to create the colour you prefer.

Skin test

It's vital to do a skin test before using any colorant as some people are allergic to ingredients such as para-dyes, which appear in many products. An allergic reaction can range from mild itching to severe burning. Hairdressers should insist on doing a skin test 24 hours before applying colorants (beware any salons that don't) and most good products for home use now include a skin test, which you must perform. A small amount of product should be applied to a clean pulse point – behind the ear or in the crook of the elbow – and left for a minimum of 24 hours to check for any bad or allergic reaction.

Permanent colours

These colorants, or tints as they are often called, lighten or darken, and can very effectively cover white. While the colour is permanent, don't forget that roots will need retouching every 4–6 weeks to keep pace with new growth.

Permanent colorant works by putting colour pigment mixed with hydrogen peroxide into the cortex (the centre) of the hair shaft during the development time. The pigment adds melanin for darker shades of brown and black, and pheomelanin for red and yellow shades.

Left The colour process can enhance the natural shine and condition of your hair, leaving it superbly healthy and attractive-looking.

After the colorant is applied, the oxygen in the developer swells the pigments in the colorant until they comprise such large molecules that they can't escape from the cortex and so are locked in.

Another way of permanently changing hair colour is by lightening it using bleach with hydrogen peroxide (to activate the bleach) to de-colour the hair, creating a very light blonde. The peroxide enters the hair shaft by means of ammonia which lifts the cuticles. Once inside, the peroxide zaps the colour pigment in the hair, making it as light as you want. It's a harsh treatment so gentle aftercare is essential. Over-bleaching will destroy the hair so be very careful. For this reason, it's wise to get a professional to do a lightening process.

Semi-permanent colours

These are more gentle than permanent colorants as there is no ammonia or hydrogen peroxide to help the pigment penetrate the cortex. Instead, while it is absorbed into the cuticle layer and into the cortex, it stays only until it is washed out. The effect can only be used to add, enrich, or darken hair colour (semi-permanents cannot make hair any lighter). The colour fades gradually, washing away over several shampoos (12–20 depending on the manufacturer and the type of hair). They are ideal for those who want to experiment but don't want to commit to a permanent change; for blending in the first grey hairs; and for conditioning hair.

Demi-permanent colours

Halfway between a permanent and a semi-permanent, demi-permanent colorant includes a small amount of hydrogen peroxide but no ammonia. It won't change the existing pigment but it will deposit more colour in the hair shaft, enhancing natural colour and covering grey. There isn't such obvious regrowth as with permanent treatments, since colour is added rather then altered, and it's kinder than permanent colour. However, it will still only last up to 20 washes.

Above There is a wide range of natural tones to choose from when you are looking for a new colour, as this colour swatch demonstrates.

Temporary colours

These are mild colorants that last about 1–5 washes, depending on the porosity of the hair. They work by coating the outside, or cuticle layer, of the hair but do not penetrate the cortex as there is no hydrogen peroxide in them. However, if the hair is damaged and the cuticle open, parts of the hair can trap colour molecules. In this case, hair must be conditioned and the cuticle smoothed before applying. Temporary colours are good for a quick change or for counteracting discoloration. They come in mousse, hairspray, setting lotion, gel, glitter dust or cream formulations.

Did you know?

- *Colouring swells the hair shaft, making fine hair appear thicker.*
- *Because colour changes the porosity of the hair it can help combat greasiness.*
- *Rich tones reflect more light and give hair a thicker appearance.*
- *Highlights give fine hair extra texture and break up the heaviness of very thick hair.*

Below Hair colour is applied via different techniques. Foils are popular and are a great way of putting fine highlights through the hair.

Below Colorants can be mixed to create virtually any shade, tone and intensity you desire. Professional colourists are true artists.

Choosing a colour

Thinking of taking the plunge for the first time and having your hair coloured? Or perhaps you're looking for a fresh new look? But what to choose? Ask friends and professionals for advice – consultations in salons are often free even if you go on to do it yourself at home.

Colouring basics

Before you have your hair coloured, there are several things you should consider:
- Think about skin tone. If you're after a natural look then you don't want something that clashes with your skin.
- When choosing a colour, a basic rule is to keep to one or two shades at each side of your original tone.
- Only have a colour change if your hair is in good condition: dry, porous hair absorbs colour too rapidly, leading to a patchy result.
- A few highlights or lowlights put through your natural colour is a good introduction to colour without heavy commitment.
- Temporary colour is a great way of testing out what you like best.
- Tone on tone is a technique to blend white hair with natural hair colour, or to blend and create evenness. It lasts 2–4 weeks and adds depth, sheen and life to hair.
- Collect pictures of hair colours you like and compare them with the hair tufts on colourists' charts.

Highlights and lowlights

These terms apply to fine to medium strands of lighter or darker colour woven through the hair. Sometimes they are applied as fine slices, especially on thicker or more curly hair. The effect can be amazing, particularly if done by a professional. Lighter pieces around the face can really open up your features and accentuate dark eyes. Adding darker pieces around the face will accentuate light eyes.

Natural dyes

Made from herbs and plants, natural dyes can provide a semi-permanent colour for highlights or lowlights, but they can't change your appearance dramatically or cover grey completely, as they generally don't penetrate the cortex.

The vibrancy and durability of these shades depends on the condition of the hair and the depth of shade you are trying to achieve. Equally the quality of the raw ingredients comes into play, combined with the porosity and natural colour of your hair.

Although henna is the most widely used natural dye, others can be extracted from a wide variety of plants, including marigold petals, cloves, rhubarb stalks and even tea leaves. Henna enhances natural highlights, making colour appear richer. It is available today as a powder, which is mixed with water to form a paste. The colour fades gradually, but frequent applications will give a stronger, longer-lasting effect. On brunette or black hair henna produces a lovely reddish glow, while lighter hair becomes a beautiful titian. Please note, however, that henna will not lighten, and it is not suitable for use on blonde hair. On hair that is more than 20 per cent grey, white, tinted, bleached or highlighted, the resultant colour will be orange!

Colouring at home

Many people choose to colour their hair at home because it is cheaper and more convenient. Today, home colorants are much improved but they are still arguably harsher on the hair and give different results from those from a salon dye. A good colouring job is also very much about where the colour is placed, which is why, if you are choosing an intricate look such as highlights, it really is best to go to a salon. If you are careful, however, an all-over tint can work well at home.

In addition to reading the instructions and following them accurately, there are some basic rules that you should follow:
- Always do a skin test first and wait 24 hours before proceeding. If you have an allergic reaction it can be painful, so don't take risks.

Left *Think about the condition of the hair before applying colour so you get the best result.*

- Never mix products from different packs, as this could cause a bad reaction.
- Keep to the times given in the instructions to avoid over-processing.
- Try semi-permanent colouring first, until you are more experienced.
- Choose colour carefully and opt for a lighter shade than you want, as many home-colour products turn out darker than indicated.
- Get someone to check you've applied the product evenly.
- Apply colour to reasonably clean but not squeaky clean hair – the natural levels of sebum will help protect your scalp.
- Use a cream or petroleum jelly around your hairline to protect your skin from absorbing colour.

White hair

If you just want to cover a few white hairs, use a temporary colour, which lasts 1–5 washes, or semi-permanent colour, which will last for 6–12 washes. Choose a tone that is similar to your natural colour. If the hair is brown, applying a warm brown colour will pick out the white areas and give lighter chestnut highlights. Alternatively, henna will give a glossy finish and produce stunning red highlights. For salt-and-pepper hair (hair with a mixed amount of white with the

natural colour), try a longer-lasting, tone-on-tone colour. These last for 20 washes and also add shine.

When hair is completely white, it can be covered with a permanent tint. With this type of colorant it is necessary to update the colour every four to six weeks, a fact that should be taken into consideration before choosing this option. Those who prefer to stay with their natural shade of white can improve on the colour by using temporary colorants such as toning shampoos, conditioners and styling products, which will remove any brassiness and add beautiful silvery tones.

Care for coloured hair

Chlorinated and salt water, perspiration, and the weather all conspire to fade coloured hair, particularly red hair. However, special haircare products are available that will help counteract fading, such as those containing ultraviolet filters that protect coloured hair from the effects of the sun. Other protective measures include rinsing the hair after swimming and using a shampoo designed for coloured hair, or those

Right For home colouring, equipping yourself with a proper colour mixing bowl and brush will make the whole job a lot easier.

Above left Colorants are fantastic at achieving all levels of cover, including 100 per cent white. Consult your salon for advice or look for products specifically designed to do this.

Above Your skin will absorb colour so wear gloves for all colour work.

that put up a barrier between the hair and chlorinated water, followed by a separate conditioner. Gently blot the hair after shampooing – never rub it vigorously as this ruffles the cuticle and can result in colour 'escaping'. Finally, use an intensive conditioning treatment at least once a month.

Colour correction

If you have been colouring your hair for some time and want to go back to your natural colour and tone, consult a professional hairdresser.

Chemical treatments

Women have always craved the ability to make their straight hair more curly or to smooth away natural waves and curl. It's possible to style hair between washes, but this requires effort so more permanent treatments are great time-savers.

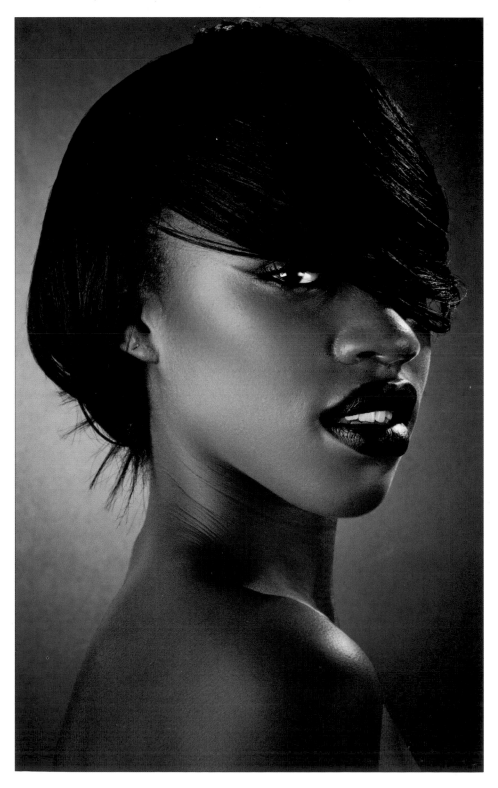

Although the way perms (for waving or curling hair) and relaxants (for straightening hair) work hasn't changed significantly over the years, they are being constantly refined and improved so they are kinder to hair. Essentially they operate by chemically altering the inner structure of the hair and re-fixing it in a different shape.

Some new products are able to scan the hair to detect variations in porosity, while others will rectify damage or loosen a perm that has been set too tight. Semi-permanent waves are also now available, and these add volume without having to commit to permanent tight curl. They can be applied all over or at the root area in particular to add lift to flat hair.

Preparation for chemical treatments

Hair should be washed prior to perming or relaxing as this causes the scales on the cuticles to rise gently, allowing the perm/relaxant lotion to enter the hair shaft more quickly. However, the scalp should not be rubbed too vigorously as this will increase sensitivity to the chemical solutions.

How do chemical treatments work?

First, either an acid-balanced or alkaline wave lotion is applied to the hair. This alters the keratin and breaks down the sulphur bonds that link the fibre-like cells in the inner layers of each hair. When these have become loose, they can be formed into a new shape, either straight or curled depending on whether the hair is stretched over a curler or a perm rod. The development time can vary according to the condition and texture of the hair.

Left Ever-advancing technology means both perming and straightening techniques are improving, becoming kinder to the hair.

When the development is complete, the changed links in the hair are re-formed into their new shape by the application of a second chemical known as the neutralizer. This contains an oxidizing agent that is effectively responsible for closing up the broken links and producing the wave, curl or straighter section – permanently.

Home versus salon

Perming and relaxing are such delicate operations that many women prefer to leave it in the hands of experienced, professional hairdressers. Although perming at home is considerably cheaper, the advantages of having hair processed in a salon are:

- The hair is first carefully analyzed to see whether it is in a fit condition to take the chemical process. Hair that is coloured, out-of-condition, or over-processed may not be suitable.

- There is a greater choice in the type of result available at a salon – different strengths of lotion and winding techniques give a range of curls that are not easily achieved at home.

Don't do it if...

- Your hair is very dry or damaged.
- You have bleached or highlighted your hair: it may be too fragile.
- The traces of an old perm still remain.
- You suffer from a scalp disorder such as eczema or have broken, irritated skin.

Different types of perm

Bear in mind the choices include:

- **Acid perms** produce highly conditioned, flexible curls with a soft curl pattern. The acid enters the hair slowly, so heat is used to speed up the process. They are gentler than alkaline perms, making them suited to hair that is fine, sensitive, fragile, damaged or tinted.

Above left You can create different results by winding hair on to rollers or bendy rods, placed either horizontally or vertically in the hair.

Above You can achieve a wide range of results using modern perming techniques, including tight curls.

- **Alkaline perms** are able to offer strong curl patterns, with a fast processing time at room temperature – no heat is required. They give striking, firm curl results on normal and resistant hair. They should not be used on more delicate or damaged hair.

- **Exothermic perms** give bouncy, resilient curls and are suitable for most hair types. 'Exothermic' refers to the gentle heat that is produced by the chemical reaction that occurs when the lotion is mixed. The heat allows the chemicals to penetrate the hair cuticle, conditioning and strengthening the hair from inside as the lotion moulds the hair into its new shape.

Above More traditional rigid curlers come in a range of sizes – often colour coded for ease of use. They are great for home or salon use.
Left Bendable rods are comfortable and great for winding the hair for a more natural looking result. Try wrapping a disposable paper around the mid-section of the rod in order to prevent lotion penetrating the covering of the rod and damaging its surface.

Home rules

If you do use a perm at home, it is essential that you read and follow the instructions supplied with the product.
▪ Remember to do a test curl to check whether your hair is suitable, and check to make certain you have enough curlers.
▪ You will probably want to enlist the help of a friend, as it's virtually impossible to curl the back sections of your own hair properly, so you'll need a helping hand.
▪ Timing is crucial – don't be tempted to remove the lotion before the time given or leave it on longer than directed.

Curl result

As with any curl (other than natural curls), the size and type depends on a number of factors:
▪ The size of the curler determines the size of the curl. Generally, the smaller the diameter, the smaller (and tighter) the curl, whereas medium to large diameter curlers tend to give a much looser effect.
▪ The strength of lotion used can make a difference, as can the texture and type of hair. Hair in good condition takes a perm better than hair in poor condition, and fine hair curls more easily than coarse hair.
▪ After a perm it takes 48 hours for the keratin in the hair to harden naturally. During this time the hair is vulnerable and must be treated with great care.

Perming techniques

Any of the types of perm listed on the preceding page can be used with different techniques to produce a number of results:
▪ **Body perms** are very soft, loose perms created by using large curlers, or sometimes rollers, to wind the hair. The result is added volume with a hint of wave and movement, rather than curls.
▪ **Root perms** add lift and volume to the root area only. They give height and fullness, and are therefore ideal for short hair that tends to go flat.
▪ **Pin curl perms** give soft, natural waves and curls, which are achieved by perming small sections of hair that have been pinned into pre-formed curls.
▪ **Stack perms** give curl and volume to one-length haircuts and are created using lots of different-sized curlers to wind the hair. The hair on top of the head is left unpermed while the middle and ends are given curl and movement.
▪ **Spiral perms** create romantic spiral curls, an effect that is produced by winding the hair around special, long curlers. The mass of curls usually makes longer hair look much thicker.
▪ **Spot perms** give support only on the area to which they are applied. For example, if the hair needs lift, the perm is applied just on the crown, creating height and volume in that area. They can also be used on the fringe (bangs) or side areas around the face.
▪ **Weave perms** involve perming certain sections of hair and leaving the rest straight to give a mixture of texture and natural-looking body and bounce, particularly on areas around the face such as the fringe.

Resist shampooing, brushing, vigorous combing, blow-drying or setting, any of which may cause it to drop.

- Once hair has been permed it remains shaped the way it has been formed, although new growth will be straight. As time goes by, the curl can soften and loosen, and if the hair is long, its weight may make the curl and the wave appear much looser.

Disappointed?

If the results of a perm are not what you expected, it could be that some of the following apply:

- **Uneven curl** Lotion was misapplied and hasn't been able to penetrate evenly. You need a salon or hairdressing professional to assess whether another perm can be applied safely.

- **Curls too tight or frizzy** Product was left on too long, or maybe an incorrect choice of curlers or rod size was used. Relax the hair by blow-drying and heavy conditioning or contact a salon to see if they can give you a curl relaxer.
- **Hair falling out in clumps** Rollers were wound too tight or the hair was combed badly in a relaxer phase. See a hairdresser – this needs professional help and you can't fix it yourself.
- **Hair meltdown** If hair loses all its elasticity as a result of over-processing it can feel very strange indeed. Avoid over-moisturizing and choose conditioners that add strength.

Below Perming the hair need not mean any loss of condition or manageability provided the right processes were followed.

Below Wait 48 hours before washing newly treated hair and ensure you use specially formulated shampoos and conditioners.

Post-treatment tips

Having done the deed, you now need to treat your hair carefully and follow a few simple rules:

- Don't wash newly-processed hair for 48 hours afterwards as any stress can cause the effect to change.
- Use specialist shampoos and conditioners formulated for chemically-treated hair. They help retain the correct moisture balance and prolong the new shape. Your hairdresser will be able to advise which you should use.
- Always use a wide-toothed comb and work from the ends upwards. Never brush the hair.
- Blot wet hair dry before styling, to prevent it stretching.
- Avoid using too much heat on fragile hair. If possible, wash, condition, then leave hair to dry naturally.
- If your perm has lost its bounce, mist it with water or try a curl reviver. These are designed to put instant volume and bounce into permed hair. They are also ideal for eliminating frizziness on naturally curly hair.
- Expect your perm or relaxed hair to last three to six months, depending on the technique and lotion used.
- Don't use metal combs or hairgrips (bobby pins) on newly relaxed hair.

Asian and Afro hair

Styling Afro or Asian hair can often be challenging. The good news is that as product formulations and the expertise of hairdressers improves, there is more technical knowledge of how to create fantastic hairstyles, whatever your hair type.

Asian hair

Usually very dark, straight and naturally shiny, Asian can be so heavy and straight that it lacks body and texture, unable to support styles requiring volume. Often to add guts, you need to turn to chemical texturizing methods including perming and body waves, although clever stylists can layer the hair to create more movement and lift. Perming just the first length of hair nearest the scalp can provide great root lift without giving unwanted curl. Adding a little colour or lightening some sections of the hair can also achieve depth and texture.

Afro hair

Often more dry, brittle and fine than other ethnic types, Afro hair needs extra hydration and care to promote healthy growth. It will most often be curly, although the degree of wave varies enormously. The reason for it being fragile is because the sebaceous glands produce insufficient sebum to moisturize the hair. In addition, because the hair is tightly curled, the sebum is unable to travel downwards to condition it naturally. If the curl forms kinks, this makes the hair thinner, and therefore weaker, at each bend.

It's vital to keep this type of hair oiled – how often will depend on the texture and your individual needs – perhaps every day, perhaps two or three times a week. Don't be tempted to reduce washing as the scalp needs regular cleansing. Do use a good moisturizing conditioner each time you shampoo. Hair that is chemically treated (permed, relaxed or coloured) in particular will need protein and moisture. Use a wide-tooth comb to avoid breaking fragile hair. Some people swear by the mantra 'condition, wash, then condition again'. Remember to rinse Afro hair very thoroughly; where detergents are not well rinsed away, you may suffer a contact reaction, the side effects of which include irritation, inflammation and dandruff.

Chemical treatments

While Asian hair can benefit from being permed to add body and movement, Afro hair can be relaxed or straightened, which is in fact perming in reverse. This process, also known as a chemical relaxing, involves chemicals being combed or worked through the hair to change the structure of the hair and to straighten it. The result is permanent, only disappearing as the hair grows.

As with all chemical treatments, relaxing, perming and colouring can be potentially harmful to the hair, removing natural moisture and leaving hair in a weakened state. For this reason it is advisable to get skilled professional help and advice.

▪ **Chemical relaxers** come in different strengths to suit different hair textures and styles. They are particularly effective on longer styles as the weight of the hair helps to maintain the straightened look. If you want to straighten your hair at home it is important to get advice first, and make sure you use high-quality, branded products and follow the instructions precisely to get the best results.

Far left Asian hair is often very dark in colour but can be lightened or coloured by lifting out the natural colour then applying new colorant.

Left Afro hair can usually be straightened very successfully using a process often referred to as 'relaxing' the hair.

• **Advanced perms** involve softening the hair by weaving it on to rollers and then neutralizing it so that the curls are permanently set into their new shape. This should be done at a salon.

To prevent frizziness and maintain the definition of curls, special lotions called curl activators and moisturizing sprays can be used to revive and preserve the formation of curls.

• **Colouring** Afro hair can be tricky to handle, because it is naturally dry and porous, so it is worth seeking professional advice when considering colouring it. If the hair has been straightened, relaxed or permed, it may be too weak to colour successfully. Techniques such as highlighting, low-lighting, or tipping the ends are best for this type of hair.

Asian hair can usually be coloured successfully but will need the dark base colour removing (or you risk orange results). This is called lifting. Once the natural colour has been lifted then it's possible to achieve the same colour results as on Caucasian hair.

Non-chemical treatments

Very curly hair can also be tamed by demi-perming. This enables tight curls to be replaced by larger, looser ones. Demi-perms are good for short hair, giving a more controlled, manageable shape, while on long hair they produce a softer, bouncier look. Made with pineapple enzyme, the treatment is good for children and those who are sensitive to chemical relaxers.

Dreadlocks, braids and weaves

• **Dreadlocks** are when sections of hair are twisted together starting a short way down the hair from the scalp. The name refers to the way the hair is locked together and can't be untwisted. Oil, such as almond oil, or wax, such as beeswax,

Far right Long, fine braids that hang away from the scalp can be worn down or up, in much the same way as non-braided hair.

Right Cornrow braids lie on the scalp and are different from plaits or braids, which hang away from the scalp.

should be applied to the hair before twisting and then the hair can be washed in mild shampoo. The only way to loosen them is to have them cut out.

• **Braids** (off-the-scalp plaits) and cornrows (on-the-scalp plaits) are a popular way to style the hair and keep it close to the head. They can be removed when you wish, although be careful not to leave them in too long or the hair will mesh together and be hard to loosen.

• **Weaves** are a type of hair extension technique that uses strands of hair attached to existing hair with specially formulated hair adhesives. This is a good method for those who want long lasting wear, from 3 to 6 months.

Special problems

Traction hair loss is caused by braiding or weaving hair too tightly. If the hair is pulled too forcibly too often, it will disrupt the hair follicles, cause scar tissue to form and ultimately result in hair loss. To help prevent this, avoid braiding or pulling the hair into tight braids. Similar problems can also result from misusing perming and relaxing chemicals. If you do experience problems it is important to consult your salon.

Above Asian hair is usually very thick, straight and glossy, and fantastic shine can often be achieved simply by combing it through.

Did you know?

Hair needs to be strong and healthy to take any type of chemical treatment. To check hair strength and natural elasticity, pluck out a hair and hold it firmly between the fingers of both hands, then pull gently. If the hair breaks with hardly any stretching, it is weak and in poor condition, in which case all chemical treatments should be avoided.

Choosing a style

Choosing a new hairstyle can be an exciting prospect. Altering the cut, colour or texture of your hair is an instant way to transform your appearance and can be such a boost to your confidence. But the choice of what to go for can be overwhelming. We've gathered ideas on short, mid-length, long and curly looks to both demonstrate the variety of looks out there and also to inspire you in your quest for a new look and a new you. Browse these galleries of headshots – whether bold and daring or more subtle and understated, there are so many ways to wear your hair. Let's go!

Shorter hair

Short hair can be the most flattering and stylish of cuts and there are many different ways to wear the look.

1 Short, textured layers give this style a fashionable finish, with just the merest suggestion of a fringe (bangs). Since it is so short, very little finishing product is required to achieve the look; it's all in the cut.

2 This striking coppery crop can be created by blow-drying hair smooth using a paddle brush, then spritzing it all over with shine spray to show off superb colour to the max.

3 Here, a deep, sweeping fringe adds individuality and drama to what is essentially a classic, round-cut short crop. A smooth, glossy finish and rich, uniform colour completes the effect.

4 Blonde shades can be stunning on short styles, but you should always ask your hairdresser for advice on what tones will suit your complexion best.

5 Bring out the texture of a short cut by applying a small amount of a soft, matte molding paste. Simply piece the paste through the mid-lengths and ends of your hair.

6 An angular perimeter gives a retro feel to this sharp, short cut. Blow-dry the hair super-smooth and add plenty of shine spray for a sleek, glossy finish.

7 This cute elfin cut is a timeless classic that is best suited to striking face shapes and clear complexions. Slightly longer layers on top can be worn smooth or textured, depending on the effect you want to achieve.

8 Add definition and contrast with low-lights of golden honey tones, which add depth and shape to a very short cut. Brushing the hair forward emphasizes great bone structure.

1

2

9

10

11

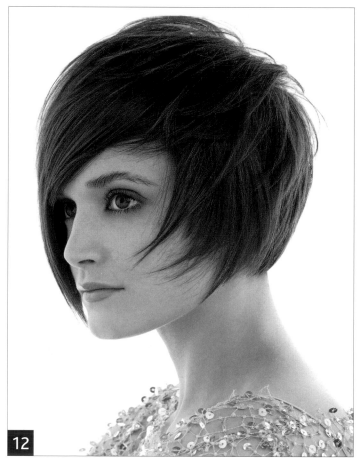

12

9 A short crop cut close in around the ears still retains the feel of plenty of movement due to texture at the crown, which can help to balance a longer face shape. Shaping or molding pastes add definition and keep the fringe (bangs) swept to one side.

10 A neat, angular jaw-length cut draws attention to a great mouth, while the strong, deep fringe helps focus attention on fantastic eyes. Emphasize great condition of the hair using a slick of finishing crème or shine spray for a glossy result.

11 Longer front sections pushed to one side are both cute and edgy. The trick here is to piece through a styling crème or light wax to hold the definition.

12 Brushing hair forward on a short cut is very stylish and shows off a jagged perimeter, which is very individual. It also frames the face and reveals a good head shape. Strong-hold finishing sprays are the key to keeping the style in place.

13 Blow-drying hair and wrapping sections round a barrel brush enhances volume and shows off the health and vitality of well-groomed hair.

14 When adding colour to a shorter cut, blending a selection of shades gives a gorgeous, natural look and enhances the texture.

15 After blow-drying cropped hair to pull it forward, piece styling wax through the front section to add definition and shine.

16 Honey blonde highlights shot through brunette tones add warmth and depth to a very simple cut. A strong perimeter shape is fantastic and accentuates full lips and strong cheek bones beautifully.

17 White-blonde hair colour can be particularly eye-catching if you have the complexion to carry it off. A deep fringe and shaped perimeter update a classic bob and create a stiking, modern look.

18 A short cut with no fringe is a versatile look – change the parting to suit your mood and using smoothing and styling products for shine and to hold in place.

19 A shattered perimeter is dramatic and stylish on a one-length cut, especially if colour is applied to bring out the sense of shape.

20 On a layered, short cut, ring the changes by tonging sections at the crown then raking through with your fingers to create texture and height to contrast with a smooth front section.

21 Leaving a section of hair to fall forward on a short round cut is eye-catching, and adds some softness and individuality on what could be a severe style.

22 When trying to grow out a short crop, go with a transition cut with graduated layers, which are short yet stylish.

23 Smooth the fringe (bangs) area on a choppy cut for contrast. Tease or back-brush the remaining areas to bring out the texture, then spray to hold.

19

20

21

22

23

24 A smooth, short cut shows off superb condition on healthy hair. Here, the fringe and side areas are connected for a very round look, which looks best on fine face shapes with delicate features.

25 Longer front sections and a higher back creates a very stylish, dramatic look. You will need confidence to pull it off, but it's a real show-stopper when you do. Keep it super-sleek for maximum effect.

26 For a more casual, tousled look on a layered short cut, first blast dry hair for texture, then tip your head forward and run your fingers through the hair for a looser, freer movement.

27 A chic, sleek bob with sharply defined perimeter is a look of timeless elegance. Blow-drying hair absolutely smooth and sleek is the ultimate way to show off a great head shape.

28 When blow-drying a joined-up bob, try pulling layers forward to show off a deep fringe area, then use styling products to define the texture and hold hair in place.

29 A very blunt fringe, longer side sections and a high, graduated back are reminiscent of the 1920s – a look that works very well with strong features. Blow-drying and tousling the back for texture brings the look bang up to date.

30 For a more glamorous and groomed finish on a short cut, push the short side sections back, then tong the crown to accentuate height.

31 On a short cut that retains some longer internal layers, blow-dry hair at the back to flick out the ends while keeping the sides smooth. It creates a more intriguing look than a traditional finish.

32 Hair with a curl or strong wave can look fantastic when cut with plenty of layering to add shape. Leave hair to dry naturally to show off the movement. Apply serum to the ends of the hair to prevent frizziness.

33 Blast-dry short hair for maximum movement and volume, then tease sections for lift. Finally smooth a single front piece to add contrast.

30

31

32

33

34

35

36

37

38

34 Wear a classic bob cut in a looser way by drying the hair smooth, then spritzing all over with flexible spray and messing up the layers using your fingers.

35 For a funky look on a very short crop, simply apply plenty of gel with a hold factor through the top layers. It adds extra vitality and strength.

36 Long layers on a bob cut are a superb way to show off a vibrant colour and great head shape. The lightest of blondes reflects fantastic shine.

37 A smooth classic bob is given an edge with a fringe worn higher than usual, showing off fantastic eyebrows.

38 For a very dramatic, upswept look, first blow-dry hair round a hairbrush to add lift at the roots, then draw hair back up to the crown and fix with plenty of strong-hold spray to accentuate the upward movement.

39 Emulate the feel of a retro quiff by backcombing longer sections at the roots and using gel and spray to hold in place.

40 For a look with real impact, keep one section of hair at the front extra long on a short crop. Crimp or tease this longer hair so that it contrasts with the smoothness of the remaining hair.

39

40

Mid-length hair

The beauty of hair that falls below the chin and sits around the shoulders is that it can be styled differently from one day to the next, and cut to suit different face shapes.

1 Shattered layers cut through a square mid-length shape with a fringe (bangs) reduce internal weight and add texture as well as showing off a strong colour.

2 Applying irons brings out the cut of a mid-length style, emphasizing the smooth connection from the fringe area to the sides. A slick of smoothing crème or spritz of shine spray is perfect to finish.

3 For interest and individuality, longer front sections are chopped into and blow-dried to flick out, creating a flattering softness around the face.

4 A choice of fiery and vibrant red tones is stunning and helps lifts a very straight-forward one-length cut to be extremely eye-catching. Be careful to use colour-saving care products to keep your new look turning heads as long as possible!

5 Fabulous auburn tones in a strongly layered cut are particularly eye-catching, showing off hair that is in great condition.

6 For a dramatic look, the perimeter of this style is cut shorter at the back than the front. A razor-sharp, exaggerated fringe adds to the style's dynamic feel.

7 Setting a parting very low makes a longer front section fall across the eye for a playful effect, while remaining hair is swept back to leave the neckline clean.

8 Pale golden blondes and defined layers put through a mid-length cut can look ethereal, especially on pale skin tones.

1

2

9

10

11

12

9 Shoulder-length hair with a fringe (bangs) can be blow-dried super-smooth, then tucked under and gripped in place at the hairline to suggest a super-wide, sleek bob.

10 On thick hair, a mid-length bob with only the suggestion of a fringe can look really gentle and feminine. Blow-dry to create volume and softness and use hairspray to hold the shape.

11 Long layers and an exaggerated cheek-length fringe section pulled over the face makes fine hair look more full and makes it easier to tame. Smoothing products help to calm flyaways.

12 Mid-length hair set on large rollers is then allowed to tumble how it pleases to conjure up a mood of effortless elegance.You can pin up longer sections to create volume and shape.

13 A volumizing mousse applied to the roots and mid-lengths before blow-drying mid-length hair helps achieve width and strength through extra root lift. Curling sections around a large-barrel hairbrush adds movement.

14 For a didn't-try-too-hard glamorous look, try tonging hair through the mid-lengths and ends, then turning under the perimeter of shoulder-length hair and pinning in place. Don't make it too clean and tease out loose ends for a free, almost candy-floss prettiness.

15 For a high-impact party look, run straightening irons over layered mid-length hair to show off the cut and wear with a low-parting so hair falls over one eye.

16 A strong, deep fringe contrasts with the shattered perimeter on a mid-length bob shape. Fine highlights are shown off through the smoother top front section.

17 A head of sleek hair is a chic look. To achieve perfection, hair is blow-dried super smooth then straightening irons applied before hair is spritzed all over with shine spray.

18 Long wispy layers add innocence and femininity to mid-length styles. This look works particularly well on fine hair.

19 For a fun, avant-garde look, hairpieces can be colour-matched with natural hair and blended to give volume and shape.

20 Set shoulder-length hair on rollers to add guts and volume, then sweep up to the crown to form a roll and grip in place.

21 Shoulder-length hair offers scope for creating strong looks. Here, the front section is backcombed and rolled to form a quiff, and the back section back-brushed for volume.

22 A close-cut mid-length bob shows off superb shine, colour and condition. Longer front sections add an individual dynamic and keep the look fresh.

23 Shattered edges on the perimeter of a bob, with graduated sides chopped into, is a modern take on a screen siren style.

24 A neat mid-length bob shape shows off great facial features and can soften a heavy or square jawline. It's perfect for showcasing statement colour, too.

25 A hidden panel of colour on long layers adds an individual touch and provides versatility on a classic cut.

19

20

21

26 To give the illusion of an elfin crop on mid-length hair, simply smooth it into a neat, low ponytail or bun. Calm flyaways with hairspray for a super-sleek finish.

27 Pinning up sections of wavy mid-length hair, rather than tying it back with a hairband (headband), creates a soft, pretty finish and showcases flawless skin. Position a mirror so you can see the back of your head to help you achieve this style.

28 A simple, neat ballerina bun can look stunning. Wear it for almost any occasion, from school or work to evening events. It is a look that opens up a petite face and shows off great eyebrows.

29 A softer take on the classic bun can be created by leaving tendrils of hair loose at the front, which helps frame the face and provides softness.

30 For a deliberately messed-up back-do, be casual as you draw hair off the face – it's a less severe look.

31 Use your fingers to rake through hair and sweep it into a chignon (twist the loose ends and pin at the back of the head). Don't worry about tendrils falling free – it's part of the charm.

32 Strong, thick mid-length hair can be cut into a layered style that is easy to look after and looks fabulous. Use a round brush to shape the hair when blow-drying and apply conditioning spray and shine spray to calm any frizz.

33 For hair with natural curl or movement, accentuate the texture by first applying curl-defining crème, then diffuse-drying the hair for a soft finish. Don't be tempted to brush it or you will create volume rather than shape.

34 A one-length bob can be encouraged to curl sweetly by tonging through the mid-lengths and ends then blending the curl, rather than leaving as ringlets, for a grown-up finish.

35 Afro hair that is relaxed can still be worn in waves, rather than having to stick to the super-straight finish. Ask your salon for advice on the best products for your hair type.

32

33

34

35

36

36 Volumizing mousse and curl-defining crème add width and texture to this style. Avoid a fringe (bangs) for a more sophisticated vibe.

37 Dark, sleek hair shines gorgeously, and when cut into layers and encouraged to wave or curl is both sultry and glamorous. Simply spritz with shine spray to calm flyaways and add gloss.

38 With clever placement, using several colour tones through the hair will pick out shine lines and make hair appear more lustrous and healthy.

39 A dramatically layered cut adds lots of texture to a style – especially on fine hair – and helps draw attention to features such as beautiful eyes and cheekbones.

40 A very long fringe can be swept across one eye and smoothed with shine cream for a great peek-a-boo effect.

Longer hair

Wearing hair to fall below the shoulders is the perfect way to show off great condition and colour. From gorgeous curl to amazing shine, the choice of looks is endless.

1 A deep fringe (bangs) adds a great individual touch to one-length longer hair. Keep it trimmed ultra-straight so it sits just above the eyes and use smoothing crème or serum to keep it looking glossy.

2 Bringing out superb depth and shine, gorgeous auburn tones are expertly applied to very long hair. With hair this long, it is essential that you maintain great condition.

3 Asian hair is usually very straight, thick and glossy, so it is perfect for a longer style. Here, a blunt, deep fringe frames the face and provides contrast with the very long lengths.

4 Darker shades on smoother hair will give maximum opportunity to create shine as light reflects better and brings out the health of the hair. When blow-drying, apply volumizing products to the roots to encourage lift in this area.

5 Simple curls tonged through the lower sections of straight hair ring the changes and add body and interest. Don't be tempted to break up the curl, leave it to fall naturally. Here, top back sections are pinned to create height.

6 A very smooth, straight fringe is contrasted with more tousled longer lengths for a groomed look that is stunning yet understated.

7 Layers cut into very long lengths help to avoid a block feel on this style, and add some sense of movement and texture. Here, contrasting extensions are used to exaggerate the length. Use shine spray to calm flyaways.

8 When blow-drying longer hair, the very ends of the hair can be wrapped around a large-barrel hairbrush to encourage them to kick out and show off front layers.

9 For a rich, luminous depth of colour, blend blonde tones from pale to darker golds and style hair in sultry waves.

10 Playing with different tones of chocolate and mahogany creates a glorious brunette finish that brings out the depth and condition of long hair. Naturally wavy hair can look good with long sections in the front, which are encouraged to sweep back off the face, adding softness to the look.

11 Long, blonde hair is a fresh and youthful look. Creating gentle curls through the front section makes a great face-framer and ups the glamour factor on long, one-length hair.

12 A zig-zag parting allows hair to sweep forward without dragging hair into two parts. It can disguise regrowth on highlights, too.

13 Blonde hair with golden tones put through can look fabulous when simply groomed smooth and sleek to show off great shine. A dab of serum keeps everything in place and looking neat.

14 Volume and texture are achieved on longer, fine hair by crimping small sections of hair, then teasing out underneath layers to create as much volume a possible.

15 Ironing the mid-lengths and ends of very long hair will emphasize the look. It's extremely important to take good care of long hair, especially on the older, more tired ends, which require regular trimming. Deep-conditioning treatments are best.

16 Body is added to thin or fine hair by having layers cut through and then applying product before blast-drying. Colour helps plump out fine hair, too.

17 On long one-length hair where there is not a style as such, have fun with high- and lowlights and add curl and wave to keep the look intriguing and beautiful.

18 For exaggerated volume and height and to open up the face, backcomb hair at the roots, then draw hair to the back of the head, smoothing top sections as you go. Apply a strong-hold spray to finish.

19 Loose blonde hair with long layers creates a casual yet pretty look. Ensure hair is tangle-free and add hairspray to the roots to add guts and volume.

20 Soft layering through the hair allows it to spring up and reveals the natural texture and colour. This is a classic look that remains sweet and feminine.

21 A fiery red colour adds a touch of magic to longer, straighter hair. With some long layers through the sides, try shaping the style so it doesn't have a parting, to allow hair to fall forward softly.

22 Avoid wearing a fringe (bangs) on a small face with a low forehead. Instead, let it fall naturally, as this will open up and balance the face.

23 Blow-dry hair wrapped around a large-barrelled brush to create soft waves in the hair, rather than curls.

24 Long hair can be tonged through the mid-lengths and curled at the ends with large-barrelled irons to create wave, volume and movement.

25 Lightly backbrush very long hair at the roots to add volume and lift, without looking like you have tried too hard.

18

19

20

21

22

23

24

25

26 Generous ringlets on extra-long hair is an archetypal romantic look. It's a theatrical alternative to a formal up-do on special occasions.

27 Thick, long hair with shorter front layers looks luxurious and full of body. It's very versatile too.

28 If you're lucky to have thick, healthy hair then enjoy the freedom of wearing it loose and not set. Simply apply serum to the ends for extra shine.

29 There's something demure about a central parting and it can be the perfect way to frame a neat face and open up the eyes.

30 On very long hair with no fringe (bangs), sections from the front can be pinned up to sit high on the crown to balance the tousled look of the longer lengths.

31 When drawing longer hair into a high ponytail, leave a side section free to help frame the face and add some softness to the look.

32 A geometric fringe becomes the focal point when the remaining longer lengths are drawn into a high ponytail at the back of the head.

33 Large sections of hair from the top and front areas of the head are twisted gently before being pinned at the crown to keep hair off the face and create height and style.

34 If you want a change from a standard, long ponytail, or need an up-do that's not overly fancy, try wrapping the lengths of the ponytail hair loosely round the tail's base, and pinning in place. Leave side pieces free to be tucked behind the ears for a symmetrical look, which adds individuality and modernity.

35 If you are feeling adventurous, try affixing contrasting coloured hairpieces (called wefts) before piling long hair up to create a truly eye-catching up-do. Remember to keep a sense of balance and proportion when creating up-dos and the results can be simply stunning.

36 Forming long hair into pigtails and curling the lengths is a casual yet pretty look. Parting the hair at the side and smoothing the top section gives a neat finish and provides a contrast to the texture of the pigtails.

37 Afro hair that has been relaxed can look superbly long, sleek and shiny. Use reputable products to take care of the hair and avoid breakage and experiment with different styles. Here a section of front hair has been drawn back over the top of the head to create the illusion of a fringe.

38 With long hair there is plenty of scope to play with contrasting textures. Here, the front section of hair is groomed to look sleek and glossy while the side ponytail is all about texture and volume. It creates a neat yet interesting style.

39 For a cute yet smart look, hair is fixed with a low parting and swept across the forehead to create the suggestion of a fringe where there is none. Pinning up back sections adds height and also introduces an element of texture for an individual touch.

40 It's tricky to dress hair yourself if you're looking for a very structured or detailed up-do. Salons will often happily help for that special occasion. Setting the hair, using padding or hairpieces, a hairdresser can conjure up very special looks to suit your face shape. The addition of hair ornaments, feathers and accessories is where the artistry comes in!

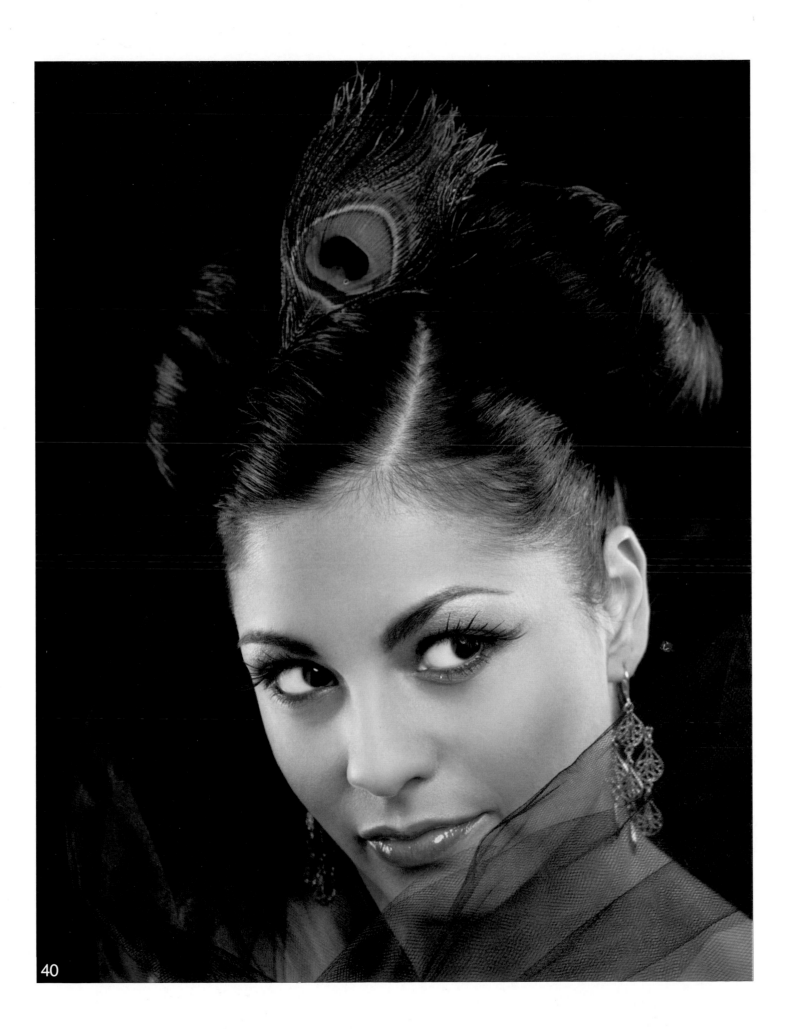

40

Curly hair

Whether you enjoy naturally curly or wavy hair or want to emulate the look when styling your hair, there are plenty of ways to work that curl!

1 Encourage wave with plenty of natural movement by applying styling lotion before rough-drying hair. Pay attention to the roots, which is where you can create volume and lift. It results in a casual yet feminine look.

2 Masses of wave on longer hair can be extremely sumptuous and elegant. Create this look by setting hair on large rollers then breaking up the curl carefully using your fingers and so as to inject superb volume into the style. Use plenty of styling lotion and spray to hold the look all party long.

3 By retaining a sense of shape and defining pieces of hair at the front, a messed-up casual style manages to be both stylish and informal.

4 Lift hair at the roots and rub defining products through the mid-lengths and ends to create maximum impact on naturally very curly hair. The trick is to create plenty of width and volume

5 Wear layered hair in a mass of curls by winding sections of hair round bendy rods and allowing to set before teasing the hair into a fabulous, individual shape. It's all about the oomph! factor.

6 Naturally curly hair still needs to be cut into a shape that allows the curl to spring up nicely and create width and volume at the crown and temple area. Use curl defining products to help style.

7 Straighter hair can be transformed by setting it on rollers or large-barrel tongs. This creates clearly defined, open ringlets, which can be twisted together to exaggerate the curl.

8 Clearly defined, fat ringlets are a head-turning look. Ensure that flyaways are calmed by using a defining curl product to smooth each ringlet, then spray to hold.

9 Use a large, round brush to create wave and movement on mid-length straight hair, focusing on the ends. Smooth and pin top sections close to the head at ear level for contrast with the wilder, more free-formed curl and to emphasize width and shape.

10 For a seductive look, contrast a long, sweeping and smooth front section with curls on the lower sections by using large-barrelled tongs on the mid-length to ends of the hair. The look to aim for is a wave rather than a curl. Very screen siren.

11 Recreate the über-glamorous look of Hollywood film stars by forming large curls with curling tongs and pinning them at the top of the head. You can work the hair so that curls at the top front are balanced with longer, loose back curls.

12 Don't brush curls as it will break them up too much and make the hair frizzy. Instead, use a wide-toothed comb on the roots to mid-lengths to create shape, then use your fingers to separate curls for better definition.

13 On longer, curly hair with no strong style, a striking choice of colour such as coppery red will provide added impact.

14 For the ultimate screen siren look, form front sections of hair into Marcel waves and spray to hold.

15 Use waves to emphasize an asymmetric hairstyle. Pin up sections of hair to create shape, then tease the ends to make them wispy and almost see-through.

16 Opt for strong waves rather than curl to create a glamorous look that also shows off great condition and superb shine on longer, darker hair.

17 Exaggerating the contrast between smooth sides and a textured, almost quiff-like top area, creates a sophisticated yet funky up-do.

18 Curling tongs can be used to conjure up exuberant volume and movement on very long hair. It's a great way to show off condition and vitality.

19 For a real bedhead look, lightly brush the surface of dry curly hair to create volume and fluffy texture. This works best on shorter curly hair, but be careful not to overdo it!

20 Using a volumizing shampoo and conditioner helps add body to a longer style. Layers cut through will help promote bounce and wave.

21 Even shorter hair can be worn in a curly style provided there is enough length to wrap sections of hair round tongs or bendy rods. The trick is to create volume.

22 Pin up lower sections of hair and grip in place to create a sense of drama with a piled-high shape. Don't make it too formal; keep it looser and fresher.

23 For a soft, stylish look, create a low parting and sweep curls to one side, pinning in place if necessary.

24 For a classic evening look, set hair on large heated rollers then backcomb the roots of the top section to create volume before smoothing over.

18

19

20

21

22

23

24

25

26

25 Longer, curly hair can be twisted and pinned to create this dramatic and rather avant-garde look. This is not a style for the faint-hearted and is more one for the professionals to create rather than something you can try at home! You can use this picture to show them what you want, however. The trick is to use padding or some support to form an exaggerated shape such as this. And plenty of pins and strong-hold spray is required to keep it in place.

26 Use false pieces of curly hair to make a quirky, eye-catching style for a night out. Colour match the pieces with the natural hair, then grip in place underneath your natural hair to conceal the join. When going for an offbeat look such as this, still remember to keep balance and proportion in mind.

27 Arrange luxurious thick hair, either naturally curly or tonged, from a centre parting into a great shape, not forgetting to apply a smoothing and defining product. It's important to keep the hair clean around the face to achieve a groomed rather than dishevelled finished effect.

28 Very tight ringlets worn in a voluminous way from a smooth top section are very dramatic. You can achieve them by setting the hair on pipe-cleaners or even forming tiny plaits (braids) and holding them between straightening irons to set the shape. Remember to set or braid hair leaving a short section of hair near the root free. You can break up underneath sections to enhance the width and volume.

29 Try combing a light gel through damp, clean hair before braiding it and leaving to set and dry. It won't create a strong curl, but will produce waves that can be loosened gently to create a soft, casual look.

30 Working Marcel waves through the front and side sections of a short, one-length bob creates a striking, retro look that complements fine features beautifully. They take time and practice to perfect but are very striking and, once you have the skill, can be versatile, too.

31

32

33

34

31 Fringes (bangs) are quite modern looking, so by wearing hair cleanly off your face you instantly evoke a retro vibe. The glorious density of dark hair colour here and the luxurious wave is very filmstar-ish in this wonderful style.

32 Tumbling curls and impeccable, sleek make-up will conjure up memories of the stars of yesteryear. It's a classic, seductive look that works especially well on a special night out. Apply defining crème to bring out the shape of the curl and a generous spritz of shine spray to work the look to the max.

33 A rich dark colour and beautifully conditioned hair looks fantastic when set on rollers and allowed to tumble free, emphasizing shine and a sense of luxury.

34 Large pin curls on longer, blonde hair is so Marilyn Monroe. Set hair, then be very careful not to break up curls when you arrange them to form the desired shape, keeping plenty of height at the forehead and crown.

35 Tonging the free ends of a loose chignon or ponytail is an easy way to give the impression of all-over curls. Use plenty of spray to fix the curls, so they won't drop too quickly.

36 Wearing hair up can look severe, so first tong or set hair to create volume and movement, then pin up sections to create a balanced shape. Allowing tendrils of hair to escape softens the look, too.

37 A true Afro look is exuberant and worked into a fantastic, even balanced shape worn clean off the face.

38 Avoid a severe or too-clean parting, or it can look as though you have tried too hard! A casual parting goes well with gentle curls.

39 Jaw-length Afro hair looks very attractive when it has been cut well so that it has a good shape. It will be easier to control, too.

40 Set mid-length or longer hair on bendy rods, then leave so the curls are more like waves yet remain unbroken, for definition.

Index

Figures in italics indicate captions.

Picture Credits

All pictures © Anness Publishing Ltd, apart from the following: t = top; b = bottom; r = right; l = left; c = centre
Babyliss 31bc.

Balmain Extensions (Hair by Steven Goldsworthy, Balmain Global Ambassador and Jason Smith, Artistic Director; photography by Jim Crone; make-up by Lucy Pook; styling by Bernard Connolly.) 75 (4), 76 (9), 86 (8, 9, 10 & 11), 87 (14, 15, 16 & 17).

Corbis 11tl (Visuals Unlimited/Corbis), 11tr (Visuals Unlimited/Corbis), 24bl (Jerome Tisne/Corbis).

Cyndy Hay (Hair by Cyndy Hay, Haze@ no. 10; photography by James Rudland; make-up by Mel.) 58 (20 & 21), 85 (7).

Hatstand Nelly (Hair by Lorraine Watson and Jan Lippe; photography by Jim Crone; make-up by Lucy Pook; styling by Bernard Connolly; hair extensions supplied by Balmain.) 58 (22), 61 (33), 63 (39).

Headquarters (Hair by Headquarters artistic team; photography by Jim Crone; make-up by Lucy Pook; styling by Bernard Connolly.) 59 (23), 62 (37).

iStockphoto 6 (Quavondo Nguyen), 9bl & 15tr (Stephanie Swartz), 9bc & 22bl (Viorika Prikhodko), 9br & 27b (Alexey Tkachenko), 12bl (Jaroslaw Wojcik), 12br (Luca di Filippo), 13 (Andrea Laurita), 14bl, 14tr, 14br (Vasiliki Varvaki), 15tl (K. Govorushchenko), 15tc (Elke Dennis), 16bl (Ross Elmi), 16bc (Jacob Wackerhausen), 17tl (Diane Diederich), 18bc (Dragan Trifunovic), 19bl (Ana Abejon), 19tr (Christine Glade), 20bc (Michael Courtney), 20br (Jim Jurica), 21tc, 23tl, 24br, 26bl (Georgina Palmer), 26tr (Paul Cowan), 28tr (Zsolt Biczó), 28br (Ron Hohenhaus), 29br (Quavondo Nguyen), 30 (Andrey Yakovlev), 31tl (Graça Victoria), 31tr (Tommy Ingberg), 33bl & 42 (Hadrian Kubasiewicz), 33bc & 38 (Matjaz Boncina), 33br & 48 (Ira Bachinskaya), 34t (Chris Bernard), 35 (Jacom Stephens), 36t (Rudolf Kotulán), 37t, 38 (Matjaz Boncina), 39tc (Eliza Snow), 39tr (Andrea Gingerich), 41tl (Ivan Mateev), 41tr (Anna Bryukhanova), 41cr, 43t, 43bl (Josh Webb), 43br (Christine Glade), 44 (Jacob Wackerhausen), 45tl (Martina Ebel), 45tr (Santino Ambrogio), 45br, 46 (Izabela Habur), 47tl (Gunther Beck), 47tr (Phil Date), 48tl (Ira Bachinskaya), 48tr (G. Powers), 49bl (S. Robertson), 49tr (Snyder), 50bl, 50br, 51tr (R. Elmi), 51bc (F. Romero), 51br, 62 (36) (K. Govorushchenko), 64 (2) (Q. Nguyen), 65 (4) (O. Ekaterincheva), 65 (6) (E. Ogan), 68 (19) (Q. Nguyen), 68 (20, 21 & 22) (K. Govorushchenko), 69 (22) (D. Tulchevska), 69 (23) (K. Kruse), 68 (19) (Q. Nguyen), 68 (20, 21 & 22) (K. Govorushchenko), 69 (22) (D. Tulchevska), 69 (23) (K. Kruse), 69 (24) (Q. Nguyen), 69 (25) (K. Kruse), 70 (26, 27, 28, 29, 30 & 31) (K. Govorushchenko), 71 (32) (L. Banks), 71 (33) (F. Camhi), 71 (34) (S. Starus), 71 (35) (J. Horrocks), 73 (37) (J. C. Justice Jr.), 73 (38) (L. Dodz), 73 (40), 75 (3) (K. Govorushchenko), 77 (12) (M. Honeycutt), 77 (13) (N. Vaclavova), 77 (16) (Q. Nguyen), 77 (17) (K. Govorushchenko), 78 (19) (J. Trenchard), 78 (20) (I. Kurhan), 79 (22) (K. Govorushchenko), 79 (23) (D. Pepin), 79 (24) (F. Backx), 79 (25) (K. Govorushchenko), 80 (26) (A. Ozerova), 80 (27 & 28) (K. Govorushchenko), 80 (29) (V. Casarsa), 82 (35 & 39) (Q. Nguyen), 82 (36) (V. Vitaly), 82 (38) (R. Christensen), 83 (40) (Q. Nguyen), 88 (18) (K. Govorushchenko), 88 (19) (M. Rzymanek) 88 (20) (F. Backx), 91 (29 & 30) (L. Dodz), 92 (31), 93 (35 & 38) (K. Govorushchenko), 93 (36) (P. Piebinga), 93 (37) (T. Marvin), 93 (40) (Q. Nguyen), 93 (38) (F. Backx).

Jo Hansford Collection
57 (14), 61 (30), 67 (13), 69 (24), 77 (15), 76 (10 & 11).

Karine Jackson (Hair by Karine Jackson; photography by Andrew O'Toole; make-up by Margaret Aston; styling by Emma Cotterill.) 55 (8), 62 (34), 75 (7), 85 (2 & 6), 87 (12 & 13), 88 (20).

KJM Salons (Hair by Kerry Mather and the creative team at KJM Salons; photography by Jim Crone; make-up by Valerie Ferreria and Lucy Pook; styling by Cora Chung and Bernard Connolly; hair extensions supplied by Balmain.) 54 (2), 55 (3 & 5), 57 (18), 65 (5), 85 (5).

Michael Barnes (Hair by Michael Barnes for The Goldwell Academy; photography by Kyoko Homma; make-up by Sabrina Ziomi.) 55 (4), 58 (19), 61 (31), 62 (35), 66 (9), 75 (6), 76 (8), 81 (30, 32 & 33).

Pat Wood for Affinage (Hair by Pat Wood for Affinage; photography by David Howard; make-up by Nora Nona; styling by Robie Spencer.) 53 (right), 57 (17), 64 (1), 67 (16), 89 (21, 22 & 23).

Rae Palmer (Hair by Rae Palmer for Rae Palmer Hairdressing; photography by Ben Cook for TIGI; make-up by Amelia Pruen for TIGI; styling by Puschka and Jiv.) 56 (11), 60 (26), 63 (40), 65 (7 & 8), 67 (17), 72 (36), 73 (39), 81 (33), 92 (32, 33 & 34).

The Colour Room (Hair by Sean and James Tetlow; photography by Trevor Leighton and Jim Crone; make-up by Chase Aston, Cheryl Phelps-Gardiner, Ali Betts and Carol Wilson; styling by Peter Breen, Desiree Lederer and Charlotte Inghram.) 53 (left and centre), 54 (1), 55 (6 & 7), 56 (9, 10 & 12), 60 (24, 27 & 28), 64 (2), 66 (10, 11 & 12), 67 (14, 15 & 18), 75 (2 & 5), 78 (18 & 21), 84 (1), 85 (3), 88 (18), 89 (24).

The Hair Advice Centre 57 (15), 74 (1).

Webster Whiteman (Darren and Lisa at Webster Whiteman.) 57 (13 & 16), 60 (25 & 29), 61 (32), 63 (38), 65 (3), 69 (22), 77 (14), 82 (34 & 37), 85 (4), 90 (25 & 26), 91 (27 & 28).